CHILD LIFE IN HOSPITALS

CHILD LIFE IN HOSPITALS

Theory and Practice

By

RICHARD H. THOMPSON, M.A.

Doctoral Candidate in Child and Family Studies
University of Wisconsin
Formerly, Consultant in Child Life
Utica College of Syracuse University, and
Child Life Specialist, Children's Health Center
Minneapolis, Minnesota

and

GENE STANFORD, Ph.D.

Director, Child Life Department
Children's Hospital of Buffalo, New York
Formerly, Associate Professor and Director
Child Life Specialist Program
Utica College of Syracuse University

With a Foreword by

Jerriann Myers Wilson, M.Ed.

Director, Child Life Department
Johns Hopkins Hospital
Baltimore, Maryland

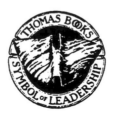

CHARLES C THOMAS • PUBLISHER
Springfield • Illinois • U.S.A.

Published and Distributed Throughout the World by
CHARLES C THOMAS • PUBLISHER
Bannerstone House
301-327 East Lawrence Avenue, Springfield, Illinois, U.S.A.

©*1981, by* CHARLES C THOMAS • PUBLISHER
ISBN 0-398-04445-4 Cloth
ISBN 0-398-04456-2 Paper
Library of Congress Catalog Card Number: 80-26935

Library of Congress Cataloging in Publication Data

Thompson, Richard Howard, 1950–
 Child life in hospitals.

 Bibliography: p.
 Includes index.
  1. Children—Hospital care.   2. Children—
Preparation for medical care.   I. Stanford, Gene,
joint author.   II. Title. [DNLM: 1. Child,
Hospitalized.   WS 105.5.H7 T475c]
RJ242.T49   362.1′1′088054   80-26935
ISBN 0-398-0445-7
ISBN 0-398-04456-2 (pbk.)

Printed in the United States of America
S-RX-1

To Our Parents

FOREWORD

The past twenty years have yielded a significant increase in the number of child life programs in North America, although there are still many pediatric settings lacking this important service for their patients. This growth and the expectation that other child life programs will be initiated underscore the need for this book.

Child Life in Hospitals presents an exciting and fresh approach to child life programming. The authors skillfully demonstrate through carefully selected case studies, pertinent bibliographical resources, and personal experience the emotional needs of the hospitalized child and his or her family, while confronting the reader with the realities of administrating a child life program.

But this book is not an activities primer, as the authors recognized that there are other resources which provide this information. They instead involve the reader in trying to understand the need for a child life program, the mechanics of establishing one, its place in the hospital hierarchy, methods of evaluating the program, and even a description of the procedure for making a cost/benefit analysis of this kind of programming. A familiarity with this knowledge increases the child life professional's political awareness of hospital administration realities.

Chapters are built on a theoretical base with thorough discussions of a variety of topics, including the elements of play, the perceptions of children, determinents of emotional upset in hospitalized children, and the importance of family involvement. The book abounds with practical aids for the child life professional. There are specific guidelines, for instance, involving the training of volunteers, the use of space, preparation techniques, effective chart notation, control of entertainment on the unit, and communication with children. Not only is this invaluable for individuals who plan to implement child life programs, but also for those eager to improve their existing programs.

It serves a greater audience than just the child life group, however. Hospital personnel of many disciplines will use this book to learn more about the field of child life as well as gather additional valuable information about the needs of hospitalized children and families. Instructors and students in the college-based programs which focus on the child life profession will find this excellent as a text for the course because of its orderly and comprehensive coverage of the subject.

Child life has made significant strides over the recent decades, not only helping children and their families experience improved care in pediatric settings but also in the evolution of the child life profession. The tools, techniques, and guidelines described by these authors make a substantial contribution to ensuring the continuation of this growth.

Jerriann Myers Wilson

CONTENTS

CHILD LIFE IN HOSPITALS

CHAPTER 1

WHAT IS A CHILD LIFE PROGRAM?

DAVID: A CHILD ENTERS THE HOSPITAL

David was an active, engaging four-year-old who lived with his parents and seven-year-old brother, Phillip, in a small second-floor flat a few short blocks from downtown. David's mother had repeatedly cautioned against running in their crowded apartment, but such warnings were apt to slip from David's mind, especially when Phillip was in pursuit.

The afternoon of the accident Phillip imagined the fleeing David to be a halfback who must be stopped before reaching the goal line of the kitchen door. David was pleased by his own speed and agility. Easily avoiding the advances of his brother, he sped toward the door, flashing a victor's smile over his shoulder. The eyes of a disappointed Phillip widened with apprehension as he watched David sprint toward an inevitable collision with his mother, who was just emerging from the kitchen with a coffee pot in her hand.

David received extensive burns to his right hand and forearm. The physician at a neighborhood clinic who treated the burns determined that they were not severe enough to warrant hospitalization. David could remain at home, but he had to return daily to the clinic for treatment. He did so for several uneventful days.

Five days after the accident, David perceived something different in the way his parents were acting. They looked very worried and held hushed conferences frequently. David wondered if they were talking about him. Were they concerned about his hand? Were they mad at him?

That evening Mother and Father called Phillip and David into the kitchen. The anxious boys took seats at the table and listened to words they did not fully understand. The family had been evicted from their apartment. They would have to leave immediately and stay with friends until new accommodations could be found. David's mother had discussed their situation with the clinic doctor, who felt it best that David be treated as an inpatient until the family was settled in a new apartment.

Late that evening, accompanied by his father and his stuffed dog, David entered the unfamiliar territory of the local hospital. He watched in withdrawn bewilderment as people he had never seen before placed a name bracelet on his wrist, weighed him, stuck his finger with a needle, and dressed him in pajamas that were not his. The frightened David

3

submitted to this treatment without protest, for fear of making the strangers even more angry with him.

To minimize the possibility of infecting his burns, David was placed in a protective isolation room near the end of a long corridor. His father was allowed in the room, but was required to wear a yellow gown over his clothing. Anxious to return to the search for a new apartment, David's father soon left.

David sat quietly on his bed, slowly surveying the room. Its pale green walls were slick and bare, except for a sink, a closet and a small window. A silent TV was mounted high on the wall in the corner of the room, but David didn't know how to operate it.

Lonely and terribly frightened, he began to cry to himself—but very softly. Perhaps if he cried too much, these strangers would become angry, and he couldn't risk that. Why was he in this place, David wondered. Was it because he had disobeyed? Would he ever find his way to his family's new home? Would he see Phillip again? After what seemed like hours of questions and worries, David fell asleep.

Through the Eyes of a Child

Every child who enters the hospital has a story such as David's. Each must leave the familiarity and security of a home setting and endure some degree of separation from family and friends. Each must submit to various procedures, some of them painful, performed by strangers. Normal patterns and routines such as meals, school, and play must be modified or abandoned.

Despite having much in common with the stories of other children's hospitalizations, David's story was obviously unique. A number of factors such as his home situation, his previous experiences, level of development, and his personal resourcefulness influenced his reactions and adjustment to the hospital setting. The circumstances surrounding David's admission to the hospital and the cognitive immaturity of his preschool mind led David to develop many misconceptions about his treatment.

The preponderance of evidence indicated to David that the purpose of this hospital experience, with its frightening machinery and oddly garbed people inflicting pain, was to punish the young offender. The logic of his thought is undeniable. He had been injured while running through the house, an act expressly forbidden by his mother. Although briefly allowed to remain at home, David suspected that all was not well with his parents. His fears that they were displeased with him were confirmed when his father took him to the strange building. There Father stood in silent approval of the pain and humiliation inflicted upon David. Ultimately, David was placed in a solitary "cell" and was abandoned by his father. True, Father had said that Mother would come in the morning, but could he really be trusted at this point?

David and the thousands of other children who annually enter the hospital develop many secret fears and fantasies, often far too scary to share with other people. Some, such as David, fear punishment or abandonment by parents, while others are more concerned about physical limitations caused by disease, or about their own mortality. The misconceptions generated by a young mind may be so ominous that they interfere with medical treatment. For example, a child who is convinced that anesthesia is a means of inducing death rather than a benign unconsciousness will understandably fight fiercely to avoid submission.

The fantasies of other children may be incapacitating, causing them to comply in an almost unnatural way with all procedures, for fear of being subjected to even worse terrors. David was viewed by the staff as a "model patient." Although he appeared withdrawn and never smiled, he was marvelously cooperative, sitting stoically through sometimes painful procedures. Such behavior may appear preferable to the angry protests of other patients, but the anger repressed during hospitalization may surface later in less desirable forms. For example, upon returning home David frequently wet the bed, cowered at the sight of strangers, and never wandered more than a few yards from his mother's side.

CHILD LIFE INTERVENTIONS

Because of the serious and long-term consequences of children's adverse emotional reactions to hospitalization and other medical encounters, health care facilities throughout North America have developed deliberate interventions to minimize the stress and anxiety experienced by children and to assure optimal growth and development. These interventions often comprise what are called *child life programs* (but which also may carry the names children's activity programs, play therapy, pediatric recreation, and child development programs).

The importance of such programming is underscored by the fact that child life services are now mandated by the American Academy of Pediatrics (1971):

There is a large and scientifically respectable body of literature which bears directly on this problem. Almost all of this literature supports the idea that the hospital experience is upsetting and that this upset extends into the post-hospital period. Therefore, it is mandatory that each pediatric service concern itself with this problem and institute specific programs to ameliorate or prevent psychologic upset in the child (p. 51).

Administrators of hospitals that are members of the National Association of Children's Hospitals and Related Institutions (NACHRI), when surveyed by McCue et al. (1978), also indicated the importance of child life programming. Eighty percent of the administrators said they consider such programs "essential" to the institution, 20 percent said they are "significant," and none marked the other response, "irrelevant."

Play programs for children were operating in hospitals as early as 1917, 1922, and 1932 (Rutkowski, 1978), but the child life movement gained its greatest momentum in the 1950s and 1960s with the pioneering work of Emma Plank in Cleveland and Mary Brooks in Philadelphia. Thus, child life programming is a relatively new phenomenon. Rutkowski (1978) in a survey of 120 child life programs in the United States found that only 18 percent of the programs had been founded prior to 1959 and that the average age of the programs surveyed was 11.35 years. The first organization of personnel engaged in child life work, the Association for the Care of Children in Hospitals (now known as the Association for the Care of Children's Health), was founded in 1967. Its *Directory of Child Life Activity Programs in North America* (1979) lists over 270 programs in the United States and Canada.

Staff for these programs come from a variety of disciplines. In surveying child life programs in the United States, Rutkowski (1978) found that 30 percent of the directors had a background in child development, 29 percent had a background in education, 15 percent in recreation, and the remainder in psychology, peditatrics, nursing, and other fields. McCue et al. (1978), in their survey of NACHRI members, found that most programs had staff with a background in recreational therapy, followed by child development and education. Mather and Glasrud (1980) surveyed programs in the U.S. and Canada and found that 20 percent of the child life workers had a background in child development, 21 percent had a background in education, and 23 percent had a background in recreational therapy, with the remainder distributed among a variety of other disciplines. They found that 59 percent of the child life workers held the Bachelor's degree. McCue et al. (1978) also found that most paid child life staff in NACHRI institutions held the Bachelor's degree. Some held the A.A. degree, but most of these personnel were working toward the Bachelor's. In approximately one-fourth of the programs, one or more of the staff held the Master's degree, and two programs had staff members with doctoral degrees.

Although these studies reveal a wide diversity of professional preparation among child life personnel, it is possible to discern a certain amount of commonality; child development seems to be at the core, with important contributions from recreation and education. Movement toward increasing standardization of the training of child life personnel is taking place (Stanford, 1980), spurred in part by the establishment of degree-granting preparation programs in colleges and universities, such as Wheelock College (Boston), Mills College (Oakland, California), Utica College (Utica, New York), Northeastern Illinois University (Chicago), Bowling Green State University (Ohio), Edgewood College (Madison, Wisconsin), and elsewhere.

The structure of individual programs varies according to such factors as size of the pediatric facility, type of patient population served, and the presence of other available services (psychology, social work, occupational therapy, and others). However all programs are guided by two primary objectives:

(1) to help the child cope with the stress and anxiety of the hospital experience

(2) to promote the child's normal growth and development while in the health care setting and after returning home.

(For a related conceptualization of the goals of child life programming, see the "Child Life Activity Study Section Position Paper" published by the Association for the Care of Children's Health, reprinted in Appendix A.)

It would be helpful to examine these two objectives individually to explore the range of activities available to the child life worker in striving to achieve each.

Coping with Stress and Anxiety

Children who are coping successfully with the stress and anxiety of the hospital experience play freely, express their feelings verbally or nonverbally, feel secure in their relationships with their families and the hospital staff, and are reasonably knowledgeable about their conditions and upcoming procedures. The child life program helps children move toward this state through the following interventions:

(1) Providing materials and guidance for play

(2) Preparing children for hospitalization, surgery, and medical procedures

(3) Lending emotional support to parents and siblings

(4) Advocating the child's point of view to hospital personnel

(5) Maintaining a receptive environment for children and their families.

Play

The major portion of children's waking lives is spent at play. It is a mechanism through which they learn, socialize, test their growing bodies, and, most importantly for hospitalized children, it is the way they cope with the unfamiliar and express their concerns.

Play is the core of the child life program. The child life worker provides abundant opportunities for children to play, encouraging them to express themselves freely in an open, nonjudgmental atmosphere. By allowing children to play in this manner, the child life worker fosters a sense of trust in children. Those children who have a secure, consistent relationship with an adult such as a child life worker will be more willing to confide in and listen to that person.

Observation of the child's play will yield clues to the child's concerns or will uncover misconceptions harbored in the child's mind. Sharing this information with other members of the health care team can lead to more sensitive treatment of the patient. A more complete discussion of play can be found in Chapters 4 and 5.

Preparation

Children need an accurate, reassuring explanation of illness, hospitalization, surgery, or other procedures, presented in a manner appropriate to their level of understanding. Children deprived of such explanations are left to formulate their own, often weaving fantasies and misguided observations into frightening inaccuracies. Thus, they may believe that injections are given to "bad" children or that a tonsillectomy revokes the gift of speech.

The child life worker seeks to assure maximum preparation of children, prior to hospitalization through preadmission visits, and during the hospital stay with explanations of upcoming events. In cases where the child life worker is unable to prepare each child, he or she acts as a resource person for those doing the preparation, advising on effective techniques for various age-groups and situations. Preparation will be discussed at greater length in Chapter 6.

Parents and Families

Children rely on their parents and families for much-needed emotional support during hospitalization. This is particularly true of children under five, for whom separation from parents may be as painful as any other source of stress. But parents who are uncomfortable in the hospital setting or immobilized by anxiety, or even guilt, over the child's condition may be less able to provide support for the uneasy child. The child life worker recognizes the needs of parents and helps them deal with their concerns —both informally, by listening thoughtfully, explaining a rule or procedure, or encouraging a parent to ask a question concerning care; and formally, by establishing parent support groups or structuring other parent programs as the need arises.

Nonhospitalized siblings are often the forgotten members of the family system. A parent's concern is focused on the ill child, often causing other children to feel neglected. The child life worker is sensitive to this situation, encouraging sibling visitation and involving siblings in the hospitalized child's play. In settings where such visitation is prohibited, the child life worker should be an advocate for the liberalization of this policy. The involvement of families in the care of hospitalized children will be discussed in detail in Chapter 3.

Environment

The architecture of the hospital, the artwork on the walls, the arrangement of furniture, the access to play areas, the content of admitting forms—all of these elements of the hospital environment convey messages to hospitalized children and their families. Children are less likely to feel threatened by a pediatric unit if, upon entering it, they immediately see children's artwork on the walls and see an inviting play area instead of unfamiliar medical equipment or critically ill patients. Parents will feel that their presence is welcomed and that they are encouraged to spend the night with their children if a parents' lounge and a place to shower are provided.

The child life worker must be acutely aware of the nonverbal messages transmitted by the hospital setting and work cooperatively with other members of the health care team to insure the positive nature of these communications. The various elements of the environment of the pediatric facility that require attention are the focus of Chapter 7.

Advocacy

Many problems encountered during a child's hospitalization might be avoided if the caregiver could view a situation from the child's perspective. Forcing a six-year-old male to remove his pajama bottoms before a tonsillectomy may reinforce a secret fear that he will be castrated during surgery. Telling a child that she will be "put to sleep" for surgery may be terrifying if she has known of ailing pets "put to sleep" by a veterinarian. Only when the staff is aware of the typical concerns of hospitalized children and of the emotionally charged nature of certain words and practices will it be possible to make appropriate changes.

Most young children lack the verbal facility to express their concerns to the staff. As mentioned earlier, children are more likely to reveal their fears and needs during a play session. The child life worker who observes a child's signal for help should respond by becoming an advocate for the child's position. For example, if a child indicates the importance of being accompanied to surgery by a stuffed animal, the child life worker should make that wish to known to the staff and work to eliminate unreasonable regulations preventing it, should they exist.

Often the child life worker will act as an advocate for the patients as a group, seeking more enlightened care for children based on knowledge of their needs. For example, the child life worker, aware that separation from parents prior to the induction of anesthesia for surgery is frightening for many children will work to change hospital policy to allow the parents to remain with their children through induction.

Promotion of Development

Hospitalization places many limitations on the normal activities of children. Bedrest is often a necessity, sometimes accompanied by traction, IV's, or other restraints. Ambulatory children may be frustrated since areas for large motor activity are frequently cramped or nonexistent. Peer contact is minimized; school-related functions are curtailed. Children who are systematically deprived of social and intellectual stimulation, particularly over the course of an extended hospitalization, may suffer a delay in the development of age-appropriate skills.

In addition to the role of facilitator of children's emotional adjustment to the medical setting, the child life worker acts as a promoter of children's normal development. Patients are provided with activities designed to stimulate growth, without causing the patients to become frustrated. The child life worker recognizes the physical limitations of patients and adapts activities accordingly. Thus, a child who must lie on her back in bed may paint on a properly-fitted over-bed easel, while another, who cannot grasp, may hold a paintbrush with the aid of Velcro™ strips.

Interaction among hospitalized children is encouraged by the child life worker so that children may continue to develop skills of social interaction. Play groups are formed among ambulatory patients. Children on bedrest are encouraged to play with roommates. Beds are moved to other rooms or to the playroom so that those on bedrest are less limited by immobility. If children must remain in the single room because they are on "isolation" or for any other reason, the child life worker should make special efforts to spend time with those children and should encourage other staff members and volunteers to do likewise.

The child life workers' knowledge of child development and their opportunities to observe patients in a relaxed play setting place them in a unique position to assess the developmental level of children. If a delay in development is noted, child life workers discuss their findings with other health care workers to develop a treatment plan suited to the child's individual needs. Implementation of the plan may be the responsibility of the child life worker or other disciplines.

RELATIONSHIPS WITH OTHER DISCIPLINES

To be successful in meeting the objectives of minimizing stress and fostering development, the child life worker must work cooperatively with other members of the health care team. Those disciplines making up the team will vary with the setting, but generally they include physicians, nurses, occupational and physical therapists, social workers, psychologists, and others.

The child life worker brings to this group a knowledge of development and of the effects of hospitalization on children, as well as observations of children's behavior gained through play sessions. Communication of this information to other team members through notes in the patients' charts, morning report, informal verbal reports, and regularly scheduled team meetings is necessary if others are to understand patients and respond to them with sensitivity.

Similarly, it is essential for the child life worker to consult with others concerning treatment plans, implications of diagnoses, family concerns, and reactions to medical procedures. For example, a social worker may have knowledge of a situation in a child's family such as an impending divorce which may provide new insights into the child's play.

Information obtained from other members of the health care team often enables the child life workers to focus their efforts more clearly. In one situation a child life worker had felt that a five-year-old male with osteomyelitis was adjusting well to his hospitalization, until a nurse described the child's reaction to the reinsertion of an IV needle. Several nurses were required to hold the child during the procedure, as he would thrash about on his bed violently, cursing his mother all the while. In response to this situation, the child life worker allowed the child to start an IV on a doll, provided aggressive play for the discharge of anger, and talked with the child about his fantasy that his mother was to blame for his condition. The comment from the nurse had enabled the child life worker to implement specific interventions to help the child cope with the stressful procedure.

Good relationships with other staff members are also important if child life workers are to function effectively in their role as advocates. An idea for the improvement of health care, though excellent, may never reach fruition if the child life worker promoting it has alienated other personnel or lacks their respect and confidence. Through personal preparedness for the position, education of others concerning the goals of the program, and responsiveness to the needs of patients and staff, the child life worker becomes a valued member of the health care team capable of initiating change.

DAVID REVISITED

Having had a cursory overview of the goals of a child life program, including its primary objectives and functions, it would be helpful to revisit young David, the four-year-old whose story opened this chapter. This time when viewing his situation, let's add a child life worker, Stephanie, and observe her as she utilizes her knowledge and skills to help David through his hospital experience.

Stephanie was working evenings the night that David arrived. The nurse assigned to David had completed an admission interview with David's father and was aware of the unusual circumstances necessitating David's admission.

Knowing that David's father would leave shortly, the nurse contacted Stephanie and briefly related the details. The nurse stated that David was very quiet and appeared frightened, although he made no protest during a routine bloodtest.

Despite the late hour, Stephanie decided that it was important to make immediate contact with David. Upon entering the room, she found David crying quietly on his bed. She quickly introduced herself, telling David that she was a person who helps children feel better about being in the hospital.

David appeared somewhat relieved when he realized that she wasn't in his room for a medical procedure, but he didn't say a word. He studied the yellow isolation gown Stephanie wore.

"I bet you wonder why I'm wearing this, David," said Stephanie, anticipating David's concern. She proceeded to explain the purpose of the gown and David's protective isolation, using language and ideas David could understand. Throughout her explanation she emphasized that the procedure was important to help David go home as soon as possible. David brightened at the idea that he might go home, for he was uncertain that he would ever rejoin his family; but he still maintained a wary silence.

Stephanie noticed a well-worn stuffed animal on the pillow next to David. "What's your friend's name, David?" she asked. For the first time David ventured a response.

"Scruffy. He's my dog."

Then Stephanie asked David how he felt about being in the hospital, and when he didn't respond, she rephrased the question to ask for Scruffy's reactions. David seized the opportunity to relate several of Scruffy's fears: he felt bad about being in the hospital, he missed his mother, and he hated the shots.

Stephanie talked with David several more minutes before she left briefly to get David some puzzles. Stephanie had created an opportunity to leave the room temporarily (getting the puzzles) so that David could see that she would return as promised. She hoped that this symbolic action would help to build a trusting relationship with David.

After returning with the puzzles and before saying goodnight to David, Stephanie assured him that she would visit again when she returned to work the following afternoon. She also mentioned that another child life worker would play with David in the morning.

Stephanie met David's nurse in the hall outside his room and related the few fears David had mentioned through his stuffed dog. After leaving a note for the morning child life worker concerning David and several other children, Stephanie went home.

David remained in the hospital for several days until his family was settled in a new apartment, located with help from the hospital social service department. During that period, Stephanie and the other child life workers implemented a program of activities to help David cope with his hospital experience.

Although David had been described as outgoing by his father in the admission interview, Stephanie and others perceived David to be very shy and withdrawn. The initial activities they planned were intended to facilitate David's self-expression and to cultivate his trust. Remembering David's willingness to express his thoughts through "Scruffy," Stephanie introduced similar types of play. With puppets provided by Stephanie, David launched into a career as an amateur puppeteer, producing many stories with themes of separation from family and fear of painful procedures. These stories provided ample opportunity for the child life workers to talk with David about his concerns. David's fears were shared with other staff members during a patient care conference, an interdisciplinary team meeting.

From a nursing representative at that meeting, Stephanie had learned that the changing of David's dressing was a particularly upsetting time for him. Stephanie obtained the necessary materials and helped David place a dressing on his stuffed dog. Since it is necessary for children to be passive and to relinquish most control during a procedure such as a dressing change, Stephanie hoped that allowing David to be the active manipulator of the materials would give him an understanding of the procedure and a sense of mastery. Although his own bandaged right hand prevented him from executing some of the finer maneuvers of the dressing change, David still maintained control, issuing orders to his willing child life assistant.

Being away from his family during this unsettled period troubled David. Several of his puppet stories told of animals who were "bad" and were sent away from home. The child life workers used these opportunities to reinforce the idea that he was not in the hospital because he had misbehaved and that he would soon rejoin his family. They felt, however, that frequent visitation from his family was important to convince David that this was true.

Stephanie, who had developed a comfortable relationship with David's mother, told her of David's feelings of abandonment and emphasized the importance of her presence to David. David's mother spent the last two nights in the hospital with David. Phillip was also encouraged to visit his brother. The child life staff felt that this was an excellent way to approximate a normal situation for David. Unlike most children who are hospitalized, David was denied a chance to interact with other patients due to his protective isolation. Properly gowned, Phillip was allowed to play with David in his room, much the same as he would at home.

Upon discharge David appeared excited, yet said good-bye to the staff with a hint of sadness, promising to visit again, but not to stay! Stephanie was pleased with this response, hoping that the efforts of the child life staff to help David deal with the scary nature of his experience had enabled him to leave the hospital emotionally, as well as physically, strong.

CHAPTER 2

REACTIONS OF CHILDREN
TO HOSPITALIZATION

The reactions of children to hospitalization vary widely in character and intensity. Consider the following example:

> Jennifer, age three, sobbed deeply and unconsolably as she followed her father down the hallway to the elevator. He tried to reassure her that he would return later in the afternoon to take her home, but this promise had little effect. A nurse had to restrain Jennifer, who struggled to enter the elevator with her father. After the elevator doors closed, Jennifer flung herself against them and continued to call for her father for several minutes thereafter.

The reactions of other children are as obvious as Jennifer's yet more hostile and aggressive in character:

> Four-year-old Calvin had been sitting sullenly in a corner of the playroom watching several children explore doctor equipment at a nearby table. Suddenly Calvin reached for a small wooden car and threw it toward the children, narrowly missing one of them. Calvin raced through the playroom door, shoving another child to the side.

Calvin and Jennifer registered acute reactions to elements of their hospital experiences, reactions which are easily detected by child life workers and other hospital staff. One can hardly overlook children who cry, fight with others, do damage to their surroundings, or violently resist medical treatment. Such reactions demand the attention and concern of pediatric personnel, but they represent only a portion of the spectrum of the behavior displayed by children during hospitalization.

Many behavioral changes are subtle and gradual, requiring a consistant, observant relationship for early detection:

> John, 15, had entered the hospital late Friday night for an emergency appendectomy. Two days after surgery John's spirits seemed as high as the volume on his radio, despite an infection at the wound site. The infection proved to be persistent, forcing John to remain in his isolation room for nearly three weeks. During this period, John joked less often with the staff, played his radio only intermittently, and read his "rock" magazines infrequently and with indifference. Each morning he would sleep a bit later. By the end of his hospitalization John was spending large amounts of his time sitting quietly in his semi-dark room with the curtains drawn.

Before three-year-old Tina entered the hospital with a broken left arm, the result of abuse by her mother, she had been potty trained and was feeding herself. By the time she was placed in a foster home on the eighth day of hospitalization, she was occasionally soiling her pants and would only feed herself liquids from a cup.

The examples considered thus far have demonstrated a few of the many reactions children display during their hospitalization. But many reactions are never witnessed by hospital personnel, surfacing only after the child has returned home. The following are examples of post-hospital reactions:

Jeremy had been hospitalized at age three for a hernia repair. The small community hospital to which he was admitted placed all surgical patients, adult and pediatric, on the same unit. Visitation was limited to a few hours in the morning and evening. The nursing staff, unaccustomed to caring for children, dealt abruptly with Jeremy, who frequently cried for his mother. Upon returning home, Jeremy had great difficulty sleeping, awakening frequently from the terror of nightmares. Several months after his discharge Jeremy showed continued reaction to his hospitalization. When in a restaurant with his parents, he began to scream uncontrollably as the waitress approached, the white of her uniform apparently reminding him of a nurse.

Tammy, 2½, was hospitalized for an extended period for uretheral reimplantation surgery. Tammy's parents lived on a farm more than three hours' drive from the hospital. The demands of the farm and the intervening distance severely limited visitation. When Tammy returned to the farm, she seemed more distant from and uninterested in her parents than prior to her hospital stay.

Sixteen-year-old Sarah made a seemingly beautiful recovery from cardiac surgery, returning home in a remarkably short time. Her parents became concerned only when she stopped associating with many friends following the hospitalization.

Rory, age six months, spent the majority of his fifth month in the hospital battling an upper respiratory infection. When he was back at home, Rory's mother observed him to be less responsive to his toys and surroundings than he had been prior to hospitalization.

The preceding are examples of in-hospital and post-hospital changes in behavior which are undesirable in nature. Obviously not every reaction to hospitalization is negative. Child life workers frequently see children making new friendships among other patients or reassuring their parents that they can manage the night in the hospital by themselves. As more sensitive treatment of hospitalized children and adolescents becomes the rule, one can expect to find more of this type of reaction. If child life programming is successful, the potentially negative event of hospitalization can be transformed into a positive growth experience for many.

Although positive reactions are possible, this chapter will focus on the undesirable class of reactions to hospitalization, seeking to answer the following questions:

(1) What are the typical adverse reactions of children and adolescents to hospitalization?
(2) How prevalent are these reactions?
(3) What elements of hospitalization cause such reactions?
(4) What can the child life worker do to minimize such reactions in children of various ages?

THE VARIETY OF REACTIONS

The cases cited in the preceding section introduced examples of the many manifestations of psychological upset hospitalized children commonly exhibit. These behaviors included crying, withdrawal, regressive behavior and acts of aggression. The range of possible negative responses to the stress of hospitalization is quite broad. Certain of the responses are *overt* or *active* responses to the situation. This category would include the following behaviors:

crying	resisting medication and/or treatment
screaming	being self-destructive
whining	being destructive of the environment
clinging to parents	fighting

A second category of reactions are the *passive* responses. Rather than making an intrusive, overt response such as fighting or crying, some children and adolescents respond as John did, by withdrawing from human interaction or giving up previously enjoyed activities. This category of responses includes the following behaviors:

excessive sleeping

decreased communication

decreased activity

decreased eating

Finally, some manifestations of psychological upset appear as changes in habits, functioning, and daily patterns. A child may suddenly develop a tic following hospitalization or wake repeatedly during the night. Many children under the pressures of hospitalization will give up newer, less well-established skills and readopt earlier, more comfortable patterns of behavior.

This *regressive* behavior can be seen in previously ambulatory children who stop walking, or in toilet-trained children who begin soiling their pants. Other reactions in this general category include:

alterations in sleeping patterns

eating too much or too little

being tense, anxious, restless

manifesting fears (of hospitals, needles, death, etc.)

being overly concerned with one's body

displaying compulsive behavior

Any of the behaviors in the above categories may appear either while the child is in the hospital or after the child has returned home. For example, children may have sleep disturbances while in the hospital, or they may only develop problems upon returning to their own bedrooms. In *The Psychological Responses of Children to Hospitalization and Illness*, a review of the literature available prior to 1965, Vernon, Foley, Sipowicz, and Schulman (1965) have drawn a distinction between "immediate responses" (behavior manifesting itself during the hospitalization) and "post-hospital responses" (p. 5). For purposes of this chapter's analysis, the same distinction will be retained. In formulating plans for the care of children in hospitals, it will be helpful to see what elements of hospitalization produce immediate psychological upset and which aspects may have longer range implications.

PREVALENCE OF PSYCHOLOGICAL UPSET RESULTING FROM HOSPITALIZATION

A significant proportion of all children who enter the hospital suffer some form of psychological upset. It is not just the unfortunate few, somehow constitutionally weaker than others, who encounter difficulties. Any child is susceptible to the traumas of a hospital stay. It is difficult, however, to cite with accuracy the percentage of children who are thus affected. As shall be demonstrated in the remainder of this chapter, the number of children suffering either immediate or post-hospital psychological upset varies according to such factors as the age of the child, the amount of information children and parents receive, and the amount of time parents spend with their children.

By reviewing the results of several of the many studies concerning the psychological responses of hospitalized children, one can gain an appreciation for the magnitude of this problem. Jessner, Blom and Waldfogel (1977) studied a group of children hospitalized for tonsillectomy and adenoidectomy. Their findings indicated that approximately 20 percent of the children studied demonstrated severe postoperative reactions. A severe reaction was characterized by "marked or persistent sequelae." Eating, sleep, and speech disturbances, tics and mannerisms, fears and regressive behavior were noted among these children, with the symptoms in some cases persisting for months or years.

The study of Prugh, Staub, Sands, Kirschbaum and Lenihan (1953), a classic in the field of hospitalized children, offers further evidence that a substantial percentage of children may suffer psychological upset as a result of hospitalization. In this study, two groups of 100 children were selected. A control group received care under the "traditional practices" of the day, while an experimental group participated in a program of psychological preparation, frequent parental visitation and special play opportunities. Although it was found that the experimental program significantly lowered both immediate and post-hospital reactions, a disturbing number of children in both groups demonstrated psychological upset. The study revealed that 92 percent of the control group and 68 percent of the experimental group displayed "significant difficulties" in coping with the stress of the hospital setting (p. 79). Three months after discharge, 58 percent of the control group children continued to exhibit "disturbing reactions of at least moderate degree," and 44 percent of the experimental group displayed such reactions (p. 85).

More recent studies show similar results. Skipper and Leonard (1968) explored the effects of providing additional information and support to mothers of hospitalized children. In their first of two experiments, the researchers found that 36 percent of the children in the control group (whose mothers had received normal hospital information) experienced unusual fear in the first week after discharge, 46 percent of the control group cried more than usual, and 68 percent had more disturbed sleep than usual. The experimental group fared much better, with 20 percent showing unusual fear, 18 percent crying more than usual, and 14 percent showing unusually disturbed sleep. The same pattern held for their second experiment. Of the children in the control group, 50 percent had unusual fears, 57 percent had increased crying, and 79 percent had greater sleep disturbance. For the experimental group in the second experiment, no children showed unusual fears, 25 percent cried more, and 25 percent had increased sleep disturbance.

Aside from demonstrating the remarkable effectiveness of communication with parents, the Skipper and Leonard study further illustrates the pervasiveness of the problem facing children who must enter the hospital. Even among the children in the experimental group, whose psychological needs were given special attention, a sizable number manifested some behavioral changes upon return home. Among the control children whose mothers received only "routine" information, the percentage of post-hospital upset is alarmingly high.

One difficulty in describing the prevalence and seriousness of psychological upset due to hospitalization is our lack of knowledge about the long-term effects. Children may readjust their sleeping patterns and, in time, reduce other behavioral manifestations of upset, yet the trauma of hospitalization may have affected them in some less obvious, but no less pernicious, way.

J. W. B. Douglas (1975) studied a group of children born in Great Britain in 1946, gaining information about these individuals, including hospitalizations, reactions, school performance, etc., at regular intervals over the course of 26 years. Douglas' purpose was to see whether hospitalization early in life would lead to disturbance in behavior or learning in adolescence. Douglas did, indeed, find such a correlation:

> This study provides strong and unexpected evidence that one admission to hospital of more than a week's duration or repeated admissions before the age of five years (in particular between six months and four years) are associated with an increased risk of behavior disturbance and poor reading in adolescence. The children who have experienced these early admissions are more troublesome out of class, more likely to be delinquent and more likely to show unstable job-patterns than those who are not admitted in the first five years (p. 476).

The findings of Douglas are partially supported by Quinton and Rutter (1975), who examined information about two groups of British children. They agreed with Douglas that *repeated* hospital admissions are significantly associated with later disturbance, but failed to find such an association for hospitalizations of one week to a month in length. They suggested, however, that their negative finding might be due to improvement in hospital conditions since 1946.

The studies of Douglas and Quinton and Rutter suggest some possible long-term effects of hospitalization; others may exist. All of the research considered thus far has confirmed that the hospitalization of a child is a serious affair the impact of which may vary from a few tears following an injection to behavioral disturbances lasting for years.

Considerable hope is also offered through these studies, for they indicate that changes in the treatment children receive have a corresponding effect on their psychological reactions. In the next section we shall examine the elements of hospitalization which influence a child's response and formulate ways the child life worker can help children of various ages cope with the experience.

ELEMENTS RELATED TO THE DEGREE
OF PSYCHOLOGICAL UPSET IN CHILDREN

A number of elements of hospitalization have been suggested as determinants of the amount of psychological upset produced in a child. Personal information about the child, i.e. age, relationship with parents, previous experiences, amount of preparation for the experience, etc., has been considered, as have conditions characterizing a hospital experience (unfamiliarity of the environment, separation from family and home, limitations on activities). In reviewing the literature, Vernon et al. (1965) found that only four of these determinants had been sufficiently investigated to warrant summary and conclusions:

(1) unfamiliarity of the hospital setting

(2) separation from parents

(3) age

(4) prehospital personality

The data regarding prehospital personality was found to provide "limited support for the hypothesis that poor prior adjustment is likely to be associated with more frequent or more severe upset both during and following hospitalization (pp. 156–157)."

The data concerning the other variables (unfamiliarity of setting, separation, and age) are much more conclusive and greatly assist the child life worker in the formulation of programming. The findings of Vernon et al. concerning these determinants, supplemented by a review of pertinent research published since 1965, will now be considered.

Unfamiliarity of Hospital Setting

Children who enter the hospital encounter many elements of *physical unfamiliarity*. They see a building that is large and heavily trafficked. They are bombarded with unusual sounds and smells, and catch glimpses of ominous machinery. Dozens of unfamiliar faces parade past the bewildered children. All of this welter of new and frightening experiences forms a striking contrast to the familiarity of the home environment. In addition, *procedural unfamiliarity* confronts the child when vital signs are taken, a blood test is administered, and dressings are changed.

One means of reducing the child's unfamiliarity with the environment and procedures is to offer a program of *psychological preparation*, systematically introducing and explaining the new elements in the environment in a manner appropriate to the age and understanding of the child. Vernon et al. (1965) offer two frequently mentioned explanations for the efficacy of preparation:

(1) Children find vague, undefined threats more upsetting than those which are known and understood

(2) Children are more upset by unexpected stress than expected stress.

The previously cited study by Prugh et al. (1953) included a comprehensive program of care for hospitalized children, comprising daily visiting periods for parents, early ambulation of patients, a special play program, and "psychological preparation for and support during potentially emotionally traumatic diagnostic or therapeutic procedures (p. 75)." The children who were treated under this program experienced fewer severe difficulties during hospitalization and in the post-hospital period than did the control group which received hospital care that was considered normal at that time.

Since Prugh and his colleagues introduced a number of different elements in the care of the experimental group, one cannot with certainty determine the amount of the improvement due solely to the preparation program. Other studies, however, cited by Vernon et al. (1965) support the belief that psychological preparation is an effective means of reducing post-hospital upset (Jackson, Winkley, Faust, Cermak, & Burtt, 1953; Vaughan, 1957; Weinick, 1958). However, these studies fail to support the effectiveness of preparation as a means of reducing upset *during* hospitalization.

The work of Wolfer and Visintainer (1975) provides impressive evidence that psychological preparation is an effective means of lessening the upset of children *during* hospitalization as well as after discharge. In this study the control group received regular care, while the children in the experimental group received special preparation and support during critical periods such as admission, before bloodtests, prior to and immediately after surgery. Basic information, sensory expectations, role identification, rehearsals, and support of the child were essential elements of the preparation process. The medium of presentation varied with the developmental levels of the children, emphasizing play techniques for younger children and more direct verbal interaction for the older.

To determine the effects of the experimental program on the children, the researchers (1) noted the behaviors of the children during four stressful events (bloodtest, preoperative injections, transport to the operating suite, and waiting in the hall of the operating suite), (2) monitored physiological conditions of the children postoperatively, and (3) had parents complete a questionnaire on their child's post-hospital behavior. Wolfer and Visintainer found:

> Children in the experimental group were significantly less upset and more cooperative than control children in all four events. They also had significantly lower ease of fluid intake rating, fewer minutes to first voiding, and lower post-hospital adjustment scores than the control group (p. 251).

Johnson, Kirchhoff, and Endress (1975) found that discrepancies between a child's expectations and the actual physical sensations experienced produce distress in the child. Children requiring removal of orthopedic casts were assigned to one of three groups. One group received information describing the sensory experience of cast removal, a second received procedural information, while a control group received no information.

The sensory group showed the least distress, significantly less than the control group.

The unfamiliarity of setting and procedures that produce upset in children also has an effect on parents. They frequently become tense and anxious, and are consequently less able to offer support to their child. Several authors contend in the so-called "contagion hypothesis" that parental anxiety is transmitted to the child, who then shows signs of distress. The Skipper and Leonard study (1968), described earlier, demonstrated that providing parents with additional information about their child's condition seemingly does reduce parental anxiety and correspondingly reduces the child's upset.

The preceding studies indicate that unfamiliarity with the hospital environment and procedures is indeed a determinant of the distress in children, and that one effective way of reducing the distress during and after hospitalization is to adequately prepare children and their parents for up-coming events. A second way of making the hospital environment less unfamiliar is, quite obviously, by changing that environment. Allowing the children to bring familiar toys from home, wear their own pajamas, play frequently, and be visited by siblings makes the hospital seem less foreign, and the child life worker should utilize means such as these to minimize the division between the hospital and home environments.

One element which has traditionally characterized the hospital environment is extreme lack of stimulation. Babies lay for days in cribs in drab rooms, being held only for feeding, diaper change, or medical treatment. Preschoolers were unnaturally confined to small rooms with little or no play opportunities. Institutionalized children who suffered stimulus deprivation over prolonged periods demonstrated profound delay in cognitive, physical, emotional, and social development (Casler, 1961).

Parental and sibling visitation, accompanied by more enlightened care by the hospital staff, has helped to eliminate much of this problem, yet it is the responsibility of the child life worker to involve all children in a program of age-appropriate stimulation. The value of such a program is indicated by Scarr-Salapatek and Williams (1973), whose stimulation program for low birth weight infants proved highly successful. In their study, an experimental group of children received systematic visual, tactile, and kinaesthetic stimulation while in the hospital, with a control group receiving "standard pediatric care," characterized by "minimum disturbance" of the infants. Testing of the infants at four weeks showed the experimental group to be developmentally more advanced than the control group, even though the opposite had been true three weeks earlier. Training of the mothers in stimulation techniques and home visitation by a child guidance social worker allowed the program to continue after discharge. After one year the experimental group had a significantly higher developmental status than the control group, nearly to normal levels.

Of all the changes that can be instituted to make the hospital less unfamiliar and more home-like, none is as important as the maximizing of contact between parents and children. In the following section another determinant of psychological upset identified by Vernon et al., separation from parents, will be discussed.

Separation

Much of the manifest upset witnessed among young children in the hospital can be attributed to the terror the child feels when separated from parents. The feeling of abandonment and helplessness in a child so dependent on parents for all of life's necessities is overwhelming. That children ages four and under display an immediate response to the crisis of separation is undisputed. This section examines the pattern of response that separation provokes and considers the post-hospital reactions attributable to separation.

Effects of Separation During Hospitalization

Much of our knowledge of the effects of separation on children in general and hospitalized children in particular comes from the work of James Robertson (1958) and John Bowlby (1960). Both authors describe a series of three stages which characterize a young child's response to separation. These phases are *protest*, *despair*, and *detachment*.

PROTEST. This initial phase may last from a few hours to a week or more. During this period of acute distress, children cry, scream, and kick, all the while eagerly looking for signs of their parents' return. As Bowlby (1960) states, the child's behavior "suggests strong expectation that she (mother) will return. Meantime he is apt to reject all alternative figures who offer to do things for him, though some children will cling desperately to a nurse (p. 90)."

DESPAIR. If the parents do not return during the period of protest, the child may enter a second stage, *despair*, a period characterized by "increasing hopelessness." Children become quiet and withdrawn, crying only intermittently. The superficial calm of this stage, following on the heels of such vehement protest, is often erroneously "presumed to indicate a diminution of distress," Bowlby indicates (1960, p. 90).

DETACHMENT. If the parents still do not return, the child may enter a final stage, *detachment*. In this phase children appear to be making a recovery, as they once again become active and interested in their surroundings. Although this may seem to be a positive sign, a problem is noted with the return of the parents. Instead of responding with behavior indicative of the normal strong attachment between young children and their parents, children who have entered the detachment stage respond to their parents with indifference. This indifference is a mechanism through which the children cope with the pain of separation. During a prolonged separation from parents, hospitalized children are cared for by a series of nurses to whom the children transiently attach. The departure of a nurse at the end of a period of care replicates the original loss of parents. Detachment is thus a defense mechanism employed by the children to cope with the loss. Bowlby (1960) states that "after a series of upsets at losing several mother figures to whom in turn he (the child) has given some trust and affection, he will gradually commit himself less and less to succeeding figures and in time will stop altogether taking the risk of attaching himself to anyone (p. 90)." It goes without saying that this condition seriously impairs the future relationship between children and their parents and may even adversely affect their ability to commit themselves to other loving relationships.

Implications of the Three-Stage Response to Separation

The three-stage process of "settling"—protest, despair, and detachment—helps to explain several commonly observed phenomena. We shall consider the following:

(1) The upset of a previously calm child upon arrival of the parents

(2) A child's greater interest in presents and material goods than in the parents upon visitation

(3) The "highly social" child who has suffered a prolonged separation

(4) The reluctance of a child to leave the hospital with the parents upon discharge.

THE UPSET CHILD. A classical argument against parent visitation in the hospital has been that a child was quite calm until the parents arrived, at which time the child became upset. It is argued that this demonstrates that the parent's visit is upsetting. In reality, such a child was most likely in the despair phase, characterized by increasing withdrawal and apathy. A visit by the parents, according to Robertson (1958), "merely brought to the surface intense grief and anger that were becoming sealed over (p. 21)." The protest by the child is in fact a positive and reassuring sign that the child has not yet slipped into the phase of detachment from parents.

THE CHILD'S INTEREST IN MATERIAL GOODS. It can be a disconcerting experience for a parent to visit a hospitalized child after a prolonged separation, expecting to receive a warm welcome, only to be met by an indifferent child, who shows far more interest in the wrapped package than in the parent who has brought it. Robertson and Bowlby ascribe such a preoccupation with toys, candy, and food to a child in the detachment phase. Children who, through prolonged separation, fail to have their emotional needs met by parents or other adults will become increasingly self-centered and will tend to develop some preoccupations.

THE "HIGHLY SOCIAL" CHILD. Three-year-old Jason had been hospitalized for burns to his right shoulder for nearly a month, during which time his mother rarely visited. Although initially apprehensive of the hospital environment, he seemingly blossomed during his third week, wandering from room to room, greeting strangers and friends with equal enthusiasm. Such a child, according to some, might be making a satisfactory adjustment to the hospital; or he also might be in the stage of detachment because of separation from his mother. Robertson (1958) contends that "this sociability is superficial and promiscuous. . . . These hospitalized (highly social) children allow human beings to come and go without regret; and, instead of being secure and attached to their parents and as full of demands as the normal young child, do not seem to care much whether they have parents or not (p. 26)."

THE CHILD RELUCTANT TO LEAVE. Occasionally the staff will observe a child who protests leaving the hospital, who clings to a nurse while parents wait to go home. This again can be seen as characteristic of a child in the detachment phase. This child shows ambivalence toward the parents and gives evidence of the tremendous disappointment felt during the separation from them.

Post-hospital Effects of Separation

The impact of a moderate to prolonged separation on the child is obvious during the hospitalization, but how do these children react upon discharge? Prugh et al. (1953), found a wide range of reactions in children upon discharge. Among younger children, those for whom separation is the greatest threat, "behavior of an infantile or demanding nature, together with greater dependence on parents" was found to persist for several months (pp. 95–96). Disturbances in feeding, sleep, and elimination patterns were noted, but generally they subsided within three months. Some of the disturbances which tended to persist were related to the child's anxiety over separation from parents and distrust that the parents would leave the child again.

Vernon et al. (1965) found that other authors agreed with Prugh et al. that most effects of separation subside within a few weeks to months following discharge:

> The available data suggest that the disturbing effects of short separation are most evident during hospitalization but that they may persist for several weeks following the experience. Long-term, traumatic sequelae appear to be much less frequent than many authors had suggested (p. 53).

Vernon goes on to note that these findings are consistent with the three-phase framework proposed by Bowlby and Robertson, since one could expect a child to remain within the phases of protest or despair during a short hospitalization. The effects of these two stages are reversible fairly quickly. Only children who reach the phase of detachment will, in theory, suffer long-term problems attributable to separation. Robertson (1958) urges those personnel involved in the care of hospitalized children to take seriously a concern for the effects of separation, despite the evidence that relatively few children develop "psychopathic or affectionless characters" through hospital separation. He indicates that "*some* children in their personality development suffer grave damage and others lesser damage from a separation experience (p. 27)." He further notes that we are relatively ignorant of the effects of separation because of our lack of "ready and reliable methods of estimating the degree of residual disturbance (p. 27)." In light of the work of Douglas (1975) and Quinton and Rutter (1976) indicating a possible link between early hospitalization and adolescent disturbances, the child life worker should heed Robertson's warning.

Quite obviously, the best way to counteract the ill effects of separation is to eliminate the separation. The child who spends large amounts of time with parents will advance no further than the phase of protest. Parents should be allowed 24-hour visitation rights, with rooming-in facilities, and should be allowed to participate in their child's care to the maximum degree possible. Chapter 3 will discuss the implementation of such policies and the role of the child life worker in encouraging interaction between hospitalized children and their families.

Age

The final variable considered to be significant in determining the degree of psychological upset in children in age. As noted in the previous section, the young child appears to be the most vulnerable to the hazards of separation from parents. This vulnerability extends to the effects of hospitalization in general. The consensus of researchers is that the child who is most susceptible to the rigors of hospitalization is the child from approximately seven months to three or four years.

Infants

It has traditionally been held that children younger than seven months enjoy a period of immunity to adverse psychological effects of hospitalization. These children do not readily distinguish parents from strangers and are less disturbed by the disappearance of their primary caretakers than they will be a few months hence. These factors decrease the effects of separation on the young infants.

Schaffer and Callender (1959) offer substantiation for the belief that young infants are less vulnerable than older infants. Evidence of psychological upset was less common among young infants (28 weeks or less) than among those 29 weeks or older. During the early period of hospitalization the older infants were found to cry more, have more feeding disturbances, be less responsive to toys and register more negative responses to observers than their younger counterparts. Similar observations were made for the final period of hospitalization, with the exceptions that there was a lesser degree of feeding disturbance and less responsiveness to observers. This latter finding might indicate that some of the children were entering the despair phase of separation.

Upon discharge the younger group of infants experienced "somatic upset" for a significantly shorter period than the older infants. Furthermore, a significantly greater proportion of the younger infants were found to demonstrate no "post-hospital syndromes."

Two other studies, Kassowitz (1958) and Levy (1960) found that young infants demonstrated less response to inoculation *prior* to the event than did older infants. This was seen as an indication of an absence of memory of previous inoculations the infants had received. From findings such as these it has been hypothesized that infants hospitalized prior to seven months will retain no memory of the experience which could be the source of later psychological upset.

Toddlers and Preschoolers

According to Prugh et al. (1953), "the child of three years and under is the most susceptible to the circumstances surrounding hospital care (p. 101)." Several explanations can be offered for the high susceptibility of children from seven months to three or four years of age. Older infants and toddlers are aware of separation from parents, but are obviously incapable of accepting explanations for its necessity. While preschoolers may be able to understand parents' explanation that they will soon return, the consolation of this message may be diluted by the child's limited concept of time, the over-riding need for parents, and the intrusion of numerous fantasies.

Preschoolers live in an egocentric world filled with magical thoughts. Their capacity to disentangle reality from their fantasies is limited. As in the case of David (Chapter 1), many young children view hospitalization as punishment. Florence Erickson (1958), in a series of play interviews with four-year-old children, found that they tended to interpret intrusive procedures such as injections and anal temperatures as hostile acts directed against them. Many children view separation from parents as abandonment or a sign of lost love (Vernon et al., 1965, p. 78).

That a young child would think such thoughts is quite understandable when one recalls the egocentrism of the preschooler, who feels that he or she is the cause of all earthly events. A significant occurrence like hospitalization, with its attendant pain and separation, looks like a form of punishment to the preschooler, one for which he or she must certainly be responsible. It is from such thinking that much of the psychological upset in young children derives.

School-Age Children

Most authorities agree that adverse reactions to hospitalization decline after the child reaches school age. Both Kassowitz (1958) and Levy (1960) noted that after about age three or four, upset before, during, and after inoculation declined. Vernon et al. (1965) concluded that "signs of psychological upset during hospitalization are relatively uncommon among children of school age (p. 102)," although the data from post-hospital upset are somewhat less convincing. Studies by Eckenhoff (1953), James (1960), Howells and Layng (1956) and Levy (1945) are cited along with Prugh et al. (1953) as offering some support for the belief that older children are less vulnerable to upset due to hospitalization.

School-age children have several advantages over preschoolers in dealing with hospitalization. They are better equipped to handle the separation accompanying the experience, and they develop relationships among other hospitalized children much more easily. Their ability to test the reality of a situation is more refined than the preschoolers', although fantasies have not entirely disappeared.

Adolescents

For adolescents hospitalization often represents a challenge to the developmental tasks of their age. During a struggle for independence from adult authority, hospitalized adolescents are asked to become dependent upon adults once again. Greatly needing the approval of their peer group, hospitalized adolescents are cut off from the group's activities and are placed in a situation very different from that of other members. Concerns about how their medical conditions may affect their appearance and their developing sexuality can create additional anxiety.

Although children from approximately seven months to three or four years appear most prone to suffer upset from hospitalization, it is obvious that each age-group has its own characteristic concerns. In the section that follows, those concerns are examined and guidelines for the efforts of the child life workers dealing with the various age-groups are suggested.

CHARACTERISTIC CONCERNS AND INTERVENTIONS FOR EACH AGE–GROUP

Young Infants

As previously discussed, it has been believed that children less than seven months of age have a greater immunity to psychological upset than children only slightly older. The studies of Kassowitz (1958) and Levy (1960) concerning reactions to inoculations indicate this, as do the findings of Schaffer and Callender (1959). Theoretical support for this position lies in observations that an infant's memory is less well developed (therefore, the infant won't remember the experience), and that the infant does not readily distinguish his or her parents from substitute caretakers, eliminating the problem of separation.

In recent years a large volume of new information has been generated concerning the remarkable capacities of newborn infants. In light of this new data concerning infant learning and attachment, child life workers and all other hospital personnel have had to reexamine the care they provide.

It has now been demonstrated that the newborn infant possesses many more abilities than previously believed. These young infants have well-developed senses which allow them to gaze upon human faces, startle at the sound of a loud noise, and, quite remarkably, to show unique response to their primary caretaker's voice. Accompanying this knowledge of the capacities of newborns is the belief that early contact between infants and parents is important in their establishing close emotional ties, or "attachment."

Kennell, Voos, and Klaus (1979) studied the effects of early contact between mothers and their first-born children. The control group of mothers and infants were allowed the limited contact which is routine in most hospitals, while the experimental mothers were given their infants for a full hour in the first two hours of life, as well as five additional hours on each successive day. At one month and at one year, experimental mothers showed closer ties to their children than the control mothers. At two years the experimental group asked more questions of their children and issued fewer commands than the control mothers. At five years the children of the experimental group had significantly higher IQ's and better language command than the control group.

This recent knowledge of newborn characteristics and development should cause hospital personnel to institute certain changes to prevent the young child from harm:

Maximize Parental Participation

Since the newborn infant has the capacity to respond uniquely to the parents, and since early contact between parents and infants may have important implications for the child's later life, the parents should be encouraged to spend as much time as possible with their infants, bathing, feeding, changing, and playing with them. In a hospital where regulations limit such contact, or where the staff is unaware of its importance, the child life worker should provide other personnel with information concerning the value of such contact and work diligently to remove all barriers preventing it.

Provide Maximum Information to Parents

Any parent whose child is hospitalized may normally display anxiety. Parents of a hospitalized newborn, particularly their first-born, can be expected to show a higher degree of anxiety, as they worry about this delicate new human. Given the keen capacities of infants, they might perceive this anxiety, causing them to become upset. Data collected by Campbell (1957) supports the idea that the "contagion hypothesis" (transmission of anxiety from parent to child) is operable for young infants. In her study two groups of infants six months of age or younger were held by their mothers prior to inoculation. One group of mothers received "fear-arousing" instructions, while the other group of mothers received informative or neutral instructions. Mothers who received the fear-arousing instructions were significantly more tense, and 47 percent of their children cried, as compared with 9 percent of the infants in the second group.

To ease the anxiety of parents, and, as a consequence, to prevent unnecessary upset to the infant, the staff should provide consistent support and information to the parents.

Provide Stimulation for the Child

A newborn infant with the capacities described above must have an opportunity to exercise and develop those capacities and abilities. In a drab room, with nothing to look at or play with, and only limited human interaction, the child finds little challenge. The benefits of a program of stimulation for infants were demonstrated by Scarr-Salapatek and Williams (1973) in their work with low birth weight infants. The child life worker should design and implement a stimulation program for young infants to insure maximum development while hospitalized.

Older Infants #5

The response of older infants to the traumas of hospitalization are generally immediate and overt. Separation from parents tends to be of great concern at this age. These children acutely feel the loss when deprived of parental support and nurturance, and register their pain with noisy, terrified protests.

The care of these children should closely parallel that of the younger infants, allowing for their developmental advancement. As with the younger infants, the child life worker should:

(1) Support maximum parental participation in care

(2) Seek maximum information and support for parents, and

(3) Provide age-appropriate stimulation for the children.

Toddlers

Children of this age are still susceptible to the problems of separation, but this trouble is compounded by other factors. The child has gained, or is in the process of gaining, skills such as ambulation, self-feeding, toilet-training, and so forth. Hospitalization often requires the child temporarily to yield some or all of these newfound skills. Children react to this demand in differing ways, as Anna Freud (1977) notes:

> Some children who have built up strong defenses against passive leanings oppose this enforced regression to the utmost, thereby becoming difficult, intractable patients; others lapse back without much opposition into the state of helpless infancy from which they had so recently emerged (p. 4).

Verbal skills are developing in the toddler, but verbal communication is still quite limited. Children of this age do, however, understand a great deal of what is said around them, even though they may not seem to be attending to the speaker. Most of the information is interpreted through their egocentric view of the world, and thus they may feel that they are the cause of events such as separation from parents or painful medical procedures.

Although hospitalization for a child of this age is a difficult experience, the efforts of the child life worker can mitigate some of the problems. In *The Emotional Care of Hospitalized Children*, Petrillo and Sanger (1980) list such efforts:

> For the toddler and young 3-year-old hospitalization is less of a devastating event when medical personnel understand the need for (1) continuity of the mother-child relationship, (2) the incorporation of familiar routines and rituals (when they are not in conflict with medical goals), (3) structure and limit setting, and (4) mastery and control (p. 221).

The child life worker should adhere to these principles through support of parent-child interaction (as is also true for younger children) and through skillful direction of the toddler's play situation. Familiar toys and modes of play from home should be part of the child's hospital play program, thereby helping to bridge the gap between hospital and home. The naturally curious toddlers should also be permitted great autonomy in play, with their explorations of the new environment being encouraged. Limits, of course, must be established and enforced to provide the toddler with a sense of security.

Because of their limited verbal abilities, toddlers will use their play as a means of communication. The child life worker, sensitive to this fact, allows children ample opportunity for expressive play and is alert to messages they transmit through play.

Children of this age are on the threshold of the period when effective preparation can be utilized. While the child alone may not be a suitable candidate for preparation, it is highly important that the parents of toddlers be adequately prepared in order to minimize the anxiety they may transmit to their children. The presence of the child during a parental preparation session is desirable, since he or she may understand a considerable amount and gain reassurance from the information. Children should be allowed to handle and explore equipment used in their care if they so desire.

To summarize, in dealing with toddlers and their parents, the child life worker should:

(1) Support maximum parental participation in care

(2) Conduct a program of play which
   (a) incorporates familiar play from home
   (b) introduces new play
   (c) allows for exploration and self-expression
   (d) has limitations

(3) Prepare the parents for the child's surgery and/or procedures, allowing for the presence and participation of the child.

Preschoolers

The child of three or four years is in the latter stage of the most vulnerable period for hospitalization. Parents are still important, and separation is often painful, but preschoolers are beginning to test their independence. Fantasies still abound for this age-group, with fears of castration and mutilation common. The view of hospitalization as a form of punishment persists, accompanied by misconceptions about medical equipment and procedures.

As with the parents of all younger children, the parents of preschoolers should be encouraged to spend as much time as possible with their child, participating fully in the child's care.

The child life worker's program of play for preschoolers should include medical play, as well as other forms of dramatic and expressive play. It is through skilled observation and encouragement of such play that many of the misconceptions so prevalent among this age-group will be revealed. Preschoolers should also have the opportunity to play in an area with other children, for they are busy working on the skill of somehow meshing their play with that of their peers.

Preparation for preschoolers is a necessity. It is important that they receive simple, reassuring explanations of forthcoming procedures, with emphasis placed on what they will see, feel, hear, smell, or taste during the event. Since abstract thought is beyond their current cognitive ability at this level, the preschoolers' information should be as concrete as possible, demonstrated with props, models, and pictures which the children may handle and manipulate. Parents, of course, should participate in the preparation sessions unless they are highly anxious or hostile. In this case, they should be prepared separately.

Thus, the child life worker's program for preschoolers should emphasize:

(1) Support of parent-child interaction

(2) A play program emphasizing expressive play and medical play and allowing for interaction with peers

(3) Thorough preparation of children and their parents.

School-Age Children

Children of school age have passed through the most vulnerable period for hospitalization. They enjoy several advantages which allow them to tolerate a period in the hospital with greater ease than they would have a few years earlier. These children are social, capable of developing relationships with the staff and other patients. Separation from parents becomes increasingly easy, reducing—though not eliminating—the necessity of parental rooming-in.

The reasoning abilities of children expand rapidly during this period, extinguishing many of the preschooler's fantasies. The child life worker must, however, remain alert for misconceptions among these children, some of which will be revealed through play and others through conversation.

One concern common among school-age children is a fear of anesthesia. Having passed through the difficult toddler/preschooler years, with the inherent struggles to gain mastery over one's own stormy emotions and bodily functions, the school-age child is highly concerned about maintaining control. Children of this age often resist anesthesia, fearing that it will supercede the control they have striven so tirelessly to achieve. Fears of death are also prevalent for these children.

School-age children should be thoroughly prepared for all surgery and procedures. Because of their advancing intellectual abilities, the material presented can be more sophisticated in nature. Parents, once again, should be included in the process.

In dealing with school-age children, the child life program should include these elements:

(1) Promotion of the parent-child relationship

(2) A wide range of play activities, including medical play

(3) Thorough preparation for children and their parents

(4) Maintaining normal routines and activities, such as schooling

Adolescents

Adolescents are an often-neglected group in the hospital, sometimes placed in adult units and at other times in pediatrics, with the decision too frequently left to the caprices of the hospital census. The most desirable arrangement for adolescents is to place them in a separate unit which is suited to their special needs. In settings where this is impractical, the staff should be aware of these special needs and deal with the adolescents in an enlightened manner.

As with the other age-groups discussed above, adolescents are trying to accomplish various developmental tasks and acquire specific skills. Whereas the infant is learning to distinguish parents from other individuals, the adolescent is working to achieve independence from parents. While the preschooler learns to play with peers, the adolescent explores sexual relationships. The adolescent is struggling for identity and considering plans for the future. Concern and insecurities about physical development are prevalent.

The event of hospitalization for adolescents compounds the difficulty of achieving their developmental tasks. In a period of increasing independence from adults, the adolescent is asked to return to dependence, to be passive and follow orders. Future plans must temporarily be put aside when confronted with surgery or a serious illness. The question of how the illness will affect sexual relationships frequently intrudes. At a critical time when identification with the peer group is all-important, the hospitalized adolescent is forced into a position uncomfortably different from that of friends.

In *The Hospitalized Adolescent*, Hofmann, Becker, and Gabriel (1976) contend that "mid-adolescence," a period from approximately 14 to 17 or 18 years, is the period when hospitalization is least well tolerated among all of adolescence. Biological maturation has been reached and concerns over sexual roles are acute. The mid-adolescent's social life, body image, and self-worth are inextricably linked to the peer group; emancipatory drives are extreme. Successful navigation through this period is a difficult enough task for the healthy adolescent. Illness and hospitalization, which directly challenge the struggle for independence and raise doubts about sexual functioning, while limiting the crucial access to peers, seriously threaten the adolescent during this volatile time.

Early and late adolescents are less bothered by the threat of hospitalization, according to Hofmann and her colleagues. The early adolescent has not reached the period of acute emancipatory drives and will be less concerned by the dependency required during the hospital experience. The late adolescent has resolved some of the issues of the mid-adolescent years, such as sexuality and independence. Relationships with parents are likely improved. Unless the illness or hospitalization potentially jeopardizes career or life-style plans, the hospitalization should prove tolerable.

The child life worker must recognize the unique situation of adolescents and provide services accordingly. As suggested previously, a separate adolescent unit should be established if possible. In any case, an adolescent lounge should be provided where teens may gather to talk, read, play music, shoot pool, prepare snacks, and work on craft projects. Mechanisms for promoting group interaction among hospitalized adolescents, such as regularly scheduled discussion groups, should be employed by the child life worker.

To maintain ties with their peer group outside the hospital, adolescents need liberal visitation privileges and adequate access to the telephone. The concerns of adolescents over their rapidly changing bodies should be recognized; maximum privacy should be afforded. In hospital settings where the care provided is not sensitive to adolescent needs, the child life worker should institute educational programs to raise the awareness of the staff and serve as an advocate for appropriate changes.

(For guidelines for working with adolescents in health care settings, see Appendix C.)

CHAPTER 3

WORKING WITH PARENTS AND FAMILIES

THE JOHNSON FAMILY GOES TO THE HOSPITAL

Five-year-old Heather Johnson entered the hospital with great trepidation. In one small fist she clutched the strap of her mother's handbag. From the other hand she dangled her beloved Raggedy-Ann. Heather perceived a tenseness in her parents which distinguished this journey from a trip to the store or an afternoon at the park. When she awoke this morning, Heather had been told to pack some of her favorite toys in the small suitcase that Father now carried. She had listened carefully as her mother explained that Heather would have to go to the hospital for a few days to "have her throat fixed," but her mother's words confused and frightened Heather. True, she had suffered through a few sore throats in the past weeks, but her throat was fine now, really! And "hospital. . . " ? Heather only knew that word as a place where old people went and sometimes died. She was awfully confused, but Heather was afraid she might anger her mother by asking too many questions.

Mrs. Johnson was, indeed, nervous. Her normally gregarious daughter, who less than a week ago had made friends with the balloon man, two softball players, and a rather large dog at the local park, was now locked in rigid silence. Mrs. Johnson had wanted to tell Heather about the hospital earlier and in more detail, but she was afraid to do so. She was uncertain of the proper choice of words or of the optimum time for preparation, and her unfamiliarity with hospital rules and regulations made her reticent to promise visits from Heather's brother, Michael, or an overnight stay by Mom or Dad. Seeing Heather's present reaction, Mrs. Johnson was certain that she had been inadequate in her efforts to help Heather deal with the hospital experience.

The atmosphere seemed all too familiar to Heather's father. He had hated hospitals since that summer nearly 30 years ago when he was struck by a car while in pursuit of a playmate's wild throw. The starched white uniforms of the nurses who passed them in the lobby reminded him of those insensitive nurses who "cared" for him as a boy. He especially hated that old nurse who had told him that he ought to "shut up and quit crying like a baby! " He had felt that it was his perfect right to cry, since he was in that hot, stuffy cast, smack in the middle of the ten-bed children's ward. Limited visitation meant that he hadn't seen his mother in three days and had no prospect of seeing her until the next weekend. Bringing Heather to the hospital rekindled those bitter memories for Mr. Johnson, mobilizing a sense of distrust. He began to question the wisdom of subjecting Heather to the tonsillectomy, fearing that she might be similarly mistreated.

IMPORTANCE OF PARENTAL INVOLVEMENT

A child, particularly one Heather's age or younger, can tap no more important resource than supportive parents. They serve as a source of strength and familiarity as the child moves from the comfortable setting of home to the unknown environment of the hospital. Parents, accustomed to their son's or daughter's limited communication skills, can interpret new experiences to the child. The presence of parents refutes a young child's fantasies of abandonment or loss of love. The hospital staff, in turn, can deal more effectively with a child if a parent is present to provide information about the child's likes, dislikes, and habits.

As with any source of great power, the power inherent in the parent-child relationship can produce positive or negative results. Those parents not immobilized by anxiety, overcome with anger, or intimidated by the foreign customs of the medical setting, can immeasurably improve their child's adjustment and minimize the potential for psychological upset. Unfortunately, too many parents respond to the event of hospitalization in much the same way as Heather's parents. Lacking information on the proper way to help their children prepare for the experience, many parents rely on their own hunch about what is best for the child. This often results in little or no information being imparted to children on the false belief that information about hospitalization will unnecessarily worry them. When a child, thus inadequately prepared, feels betrayed and reacts to parents with anger and distrust, the parents may consequently develop feelings of guilt over their failure.

Other parents, such as Heather's father, harbor feelings of hostility toward medical personnel generated by unfortunate past experiences. Children who observe their parents reacting to the hospital staff with suspicion can hardly develop their own sense of confidence in the treatment they receive.

The discomfort, anxiety or guilt that a parent might feel in a hospital environment will be readily perceived by the child. Children may register a corresponding increase in anxiety, become less cooperative, or manifest other behavior indicative of psychological upset. Despite the possibility of problems arising from the parent-child relationship, it is imperative that parents be maximally included in the child's hospitalization. The potential benefit from the parents' presence is so vast, and the horrors of their absence so well-documented, that excluding or severely limiting their participation is unthinkable.

The challenge to the child life worker and all other pediatric health care professionals is to provide parents with the structure, information and support necessary to enable them to assist their children through this difficult period. In a setting where child-parent interaction is limited by hospital regulations, the child life worker must be prepared to accept the role of advocate for liberal visitation and rooming-in policies. Visitation by siblings should also be endorsed, for the hospitalization of one child represents a disruption in the life of all children in a family. Nonhospitalized siblings are also in need of parental presence and support, and the child life worker should be sensitive to this fact and include these children in child life programming.

When the parents' right to open visitation and rooming-in has been established, the efforts of child life workers and other concerned health care personnel must refocus on the effective organization of a family-child care program. Basic "ground-rules" must be established and areas of potential conflict examined. Anticipation of possible sources of trouble, coupled with swift, judicious action to eliminate them will help to defuse criticism of the program.

The child life worker also helps to establish and maintain an open line of communication with the family of the hospitalized child. Beginning with the preadmission tour and continuing through preparation sessions, parent meetings, and informal contacts, the child life staff offers information and support to the parents. Parents who feel comfortable in the hospital environment and who feel that their presence is not merely tolerated but encouraged are most capable of helping their children cope with the traumas of hospitalization.

The present chapter will deal with the above-mentioned obligations of the child life worker to the family of the hospitalized child, concentrating on the following aspects:

(1) Advocacy for an expanded family role

(2) Establishment of rooming-in programs

(3) Types of information and support necessary for all parents

ADVOCACY FOR AN EXPANDED FAMILY ROLE

Despite the massive body of literature generated since the mid-1940s detailing the difficulties of hospitalized children when separated from their parents, hospitals have demonstrated plodding reluctance to admit parents as full partners in the care of their children. For years parental visitation was limited to a few hours per week in most settings. The thought of a parent rooming-in with a child was practically inconceivable. Although this situation has improved in recent years, with more facilities increasing their visiting hours or allowing 24-hour parental visitation and rooming-in, an unfortunate number of hospitals lag behind.

Some have maintained limited visiting hours "on the books" and posted near the entrances, but claim that they don't really bother to enforce the regulations anyway—overlooking the fact that parents have no way of knowing that the rules are not generally enforced and that many parents are probably being kept away from their children by the rules.

But even in hospitals that do officially grant parents unrestricted visitation and rooming-in privileges, parents may not be welcomed. In a study conducted by Hardgrove (1980), hospitals that had previously indicated that they were committed to including parents and that they offered accommodations for parents were queried about the steps they take to assure that parents are not merely tolerated but welcomed. She found that

> ... institutional support of parental presence (in hospitals that allow it) is, for the most part, limited to providing beds. Accommodations such as bathing space reserved for parents, kitchen and meeting rooms were uncommon. Psychological support, too, on an organized basis was limited. Only 8 percent of the hospitals surveyed had a parent advocate employed whose concern it is to look after parents and coordinate their care. Only 6 percent had a place for parents to cook. Only 11 percent supplied meals at no cost to parents (p. 221).

Hardgrove also found that little attention was given to preparing parents before hospitalization and little support was offered during hospitalization.

Thus, even though hospital regulations may permit parents to stay with their children, if they are not informed of their right to stay and if nothing is provided for their comfort other than a straight-back chair, parents may be deterred from doing so. Other means of discouraging parental visitation exist which make the parents feel that their permission to remain hangs by a tenuous thread. A hospital in Utica, New York, for example, issued an information sheet to parents which introduced the new liberalized 24-hour visitation policy. Parents were advised that this policy was being tried experimentally and would be revoked should parents abuse this "privilege" or fail to abide by the rules. The message given parents under such conditions is not "You are welcome here," but rather, "Watch your step!" While, certainly, guidelines are helpful in facilitating parents' adjustment to the hospital, it is not helpful to either parents or patients to imply that access to their children is a privilege that will be quickly revoked if parents don't please the staff. (By contrast, I.W.K. Hospital for Children in Halifax, Nova Scotia, opens their statement of visitation policy with a declaration to the effect that "Since we do not consider parents to be visitors, they are welcome to stay with their child around the clock." At this hospital, 24-hour visitation is clearly seen as the parents' right, not a privilege.)

Visitation of siblings and other young children is frequently prohibited, even among the more progressive institutions which allow expanded parental involvement. Such a policy demonstrates insensitivity and inconsistency in identifying the needs of the family. Parents may, on the one hand, be encouraged to spend more time at the hospital, but if siblings cannot be included in the activities of the hospitalized child, parents may increasingly neglect unhospitalized siblings. Such a situation unnecessarily increases the strain on the family unit.

Child life workers who find themselves in institutions which prohibit 24-hour parental visitation, rooming-in by parents, or sibling visitation should be prepared to adopt the role of advocate seeking revision of these policies. A working knowledge of the theoretical arguments in support of such policies will help child life workers present a convincing case for the necessity for change:

Effects of Separation

The most convincing argument in support of the presence of parents lies in the effects of separation from parents on the hospitalized child. As discussed in the preceding chapter, children separated from their parents for hospitalization endure a period of great anguish. The early period of "protest," characterized by the cries and screams of the child, may slip into the potentially more devastating periods of "despair" and "detachment" if they are uninterrupted by parental visitation. By encouraging parents to visit frequently and to stay overnight with their young children, the hospital staff can prevent much of the child's immediate suffering and minimize the post-hospital problems which commonly affect children.

Aside from the prevention of psychological distress, parental involvement has many other positive influences on the successful treatment of the child. Parents have a great deal of knowledge about the habits of their children which can aid the staff in its efforts to care for the ill child. Information concerning favorite foods, sleep habits and particular fears of the child permit more sensitive care. Parents can more easily communicate with their children than can staff people less fluent in the child's unique language. The proper word from a trusted parent can assure the child that the nurse is, in fact, bringing lunch rather than more medicine. If the nurse alone were to attempt to convince the child, the result might well be a terrified, hungry child.

Stress on the Family

The child who enters the hospital is a part of a family system. If the child is part of a strong, functional family and if the hospitalization is relatively brief and the illness not too serious, the family may weather the crisis with few ill effects. But families in other situations may not fare so well. A family which is functioning poorly, torn apart by anger and dissension or experiencing grave problems in communication, may not be able to cope with a relatively minor hospitalization. A highly functional family, when suddenly faced with extraordinary circumstances such as the birth of a defective child or the diagnosis of a leukemic child, may have difficulty coping with the situation. Family disintegration may result. Only by inviting the family into the hospital setting is it possible to observe the viability of the family structure and its adaptation to the crisis. When problems are detected, appropriate interventions can be implemented. If the family's access to the child is limited, the child life worker and other personnel will have less opportunity to assess the family's coping abilities. Also, since limited presence at the hospital hampers development of trusting parent-staff relationships, parents may be less receptive to interventions suggested by the staff.

Although any illness or hospitalization may place a severe stress on the family system, chronic conditions present their own special hazards. Burton (1975) discusses a number of these concerns in her study of children with cystic fibrosis and their families. Many parents react to the illness of their child with feelings of guilt, believing that there was something they might have done to prevent their child's misfortune. In the case of a genetically inherited disease such as cystic fibrosis, such feelings reach their peak. Chronic conditions also by their very nature force changes on the life-style of the family, which can lead to parental resentment and financial hardship. If the chronically ill child requires frequent specialized treatment, the family may be forced to move from a distant location closer to the health care center. Financial difficulties may arise due to the high cost of medical care and special equipment used in the treatment of the child. Parents may be forced to move from lower paying, more satisfying work to higher paying jobs, or to take a second job, in order to meet hospital costs.

Children who must not only struggle against a chronic medical condition, but also face increased family tensions arising from problems associated with that condition find themselves in an extremely difficult situation. Encouraging parents to come to the hospital with their children allows the hospital staff to monitor the progress of the family as it attempts to cope with its situation. The hospital staff offer necessary support to the parents so that they will be better able to help their children to handle the difficulties presented by the illness.

Similar to the chronic condition is the birth and subsequent hospitalization of a defective child. For months the parents planned for and awaited the birth of their infant, assuming that it would be healthy and sound. When that idealized child is not born, the parents mourn the loss of the child that might have been. Here again, the supreme support and understanding of the hospital personnel are required to help the parents cope with their feelings. At the same time the staff must be concerned about the parent-child bonding process, which may now be severely hampered. Parental attempts to bond to a physically unattractive or constitutionally weak infant may be a difficult enough task; hospital regulations which severely restrict parent-infant contact, or attitudes which make the parents feel less than welcome can only frustrate this important process.

By sincerely welcoming parents as partners in care of their children, the hospital staff can assure greater presence of the parents. This not only allows the staff to support the family and hopefully avoid family disintegration, but it also provides for detection of problems based within the family system. For example, a child life worker's observation that an asthmatic child's breathing became increasingly labored after witnessing a fight between her parents helped to pinpoint a source of stress triggering the child's attacks. Allowing the child to return to her home environment without providing help to reduce some of the family's stress would condemn the child to repeated hospital admissions.

A truly comprehensive concern for the health of children includes an understanding of their family life. To minister to the physical needs of children while ignoring their social context is to provide inadequate health care. By working closely with the families of hospitalized children child life workers and all other hospital personnel can watch for signs of stress which either arise from or aggravate the illness of the child. Parents who are not welcomed and—to use Hardgrove's word—"courted" by the hospital staff may remain away, thus retarding an important aspect of the care of their children.

Sibling Involvement

Nonhospitalized children have no special immunity to the difficulties experienced by parents and the hospitalized sibling. These children suffer the pain of separation when parents spend prolonged periods at the hospital. They must often endure periods of increased parental irritability engendered by concern over the illness of another child. The emotional and economic resources of the family may be concentrated on the hospitalized child, creating at least temporary neglect of the other children. Despite the stresses to which these children may be subjected, official hospital policy too often prevents their visitation, excluding them from the hospital experience. While the physical needs of the hospitalized child may be met, as may the emotional needs of the parents in the hospital setting, exclusion of nonhospitalized siblings may create another set of stress-producing problems with which the family must deal.

The encouragement of sibling visitation produces a number of positive results, perhaps chief of which is normalization of the experience of hospitalization for all children. As discussed in Chapter 2, an important way of reducing the stress of hospitalization is to make the setting less foreign. The institution of sibling visitation can foster this condition.

Hospitalized children who are permitted access to their siblings feel less isolated, less abandoned than if such visitation is proscribed. Children in the hospital can better monitor the home situation and dispel fantasies that they have been replaced when they have a chance to "compare notes" with their siblings and to actually interact with the family as a whole unit.

In a similar manner this visitation helps to normalize the generally disrupting event of hospitalization for the nonhospitalized child. Instead of being subjected to frequent or prolonged periods of separation from parents while they visit at the hospital, the sibling can go along and be a part of the experience. Frequently when children are denied the right of visitation of their siblings, they develop fantasies about the hospitalized sibling's condition. A child's acting-out in school or behavioral disturbances at home may, for example, be linked to a belief that the hospitalized sibling is dead and that the parents' story about hospitalization is untrue. Contact with the hospitalized child can help minimize such fantasies and the problems caused by them.

In some cases siblings may indeed have cause to worry about the hospitalized child. The critical illness of a child, a newly diagnosed chronic condition or physical disabilities caused by an accident may drastically affect the life-style of the family, including the other children. Adaptation to the child's new condition by the unaffected sibling may take several forms. Burton (1975) noted that the reactions of siblings of children with cystic fibrosis tended to depend on the relative ages of the children. Siblings older than the afflicted child tended to become more protective and caring. While these older children might resent the increased attention the parents gave the child with cystic fibrosis, they seemed better able to appreciate its necessity. Siblings younger than the ill child tended not to respond to the illness directly, reacting rather with jealousy to the extra attention now focused on the other child.

Barring children from hospital visitation confounds the adaptation process. Children hospitalized for a prolonged condition who have older siblings may be denied the additional support demonstrated by the siblings of cystic fibrosis patients, if visitation has not been extended to all family members. The feelings of jealousy noted in younger siblings can only be heightened by exclusion from participation in family visits. If sibling visitation is not allowed, hospital personnel have no opportunity to observe the adaptive processes of the other children. Thus, they are less able to provide parents with much-needed advice and support in dealing with their children's reactions.

Even as hospitalized children and their parents need adequate explanations of illnesses and hospital procedures, so do siblings. Imperfect or inadequate knowledge of a sibling's condition can unnecessarily lead to upset. Unfortunately, parents all too often neglect to provide siblings with information concerning the child in the hospital, causing the children at home to spin fantasies to fill the void. Burton (1975) found that 53 percent of the parents in her study never mentioned the child's illness to the other children. Many parents expressed a discomfort in discussing this information with their children, which was apparently perceived by the children, who thereupon entered into a "conspiracy of silence" with the parents. Only 43 percent of the mothers and 27 percent of the fathers were asked about cystic fibrosis by the well children. By allowing siblings to visit hospitalized children, hospital staff can provide important information about the health and treatment of the hospitalized child, information which they might otherwise be denied. Siblings should be allowed to take part in preadmission tours and in-hospital preparation sessions. Further information can be obtained through informal contacts with hospital personnel and through the child's own observation of routines. In addition to improving understanding of the hospitalized child's situation, visitation allows children to become more familiar with the hospital environment. This familiarity will prove valuable should they themselves later require hospitalization.

Aside from the psychological advantage of permitting sibling visitation, an important practical consideration exists. Many parents, particularly single parents, find it difficult to arrange for supervision of nonhospitalized children when planning to visit the hospital. Such parents are placed in an awkward dilemma. To visit the hospitalized child, other siblings must be neglected; to properly supervise the siblings, hospital visitation must be curtailed. Hospital policy can demonstrate a recognition of this problem and a commitment to the importance of parental visitation by welcoming siblings to the hospital and by extending to them services, such as supervised play experiences.

Common Objections to Family Visitation

Despite the knowledge that parental rooming-in and liberal family visitation ease the problems of separation and aid in the reduction and management of family stress, many institutions persist in limiting visitation and banning young siblings. Rooming-in may be allowed by official policy, while parents are unofficially discouraged from taking advantage of it. Much of the resistance to these policies is based on old myths and mistaken notions, which child life workers and other concerned professionals must dispel.

Myth 1: Parent Visitation Upsets Children

As noted in the preceding chapter, hospital staff often argue against parental visitation saying that it produces upset in the children. One rebuttal to this argument is offered by Robertson (1958), who contends that the cries of children upon reuniting with their parents are, in fact, positive in nature, indicating that the child's attachment to parents is still strong despite the period of separation. An absence of crying, while perhaps more tolerable from the point of view of the staff, may be evidence of the child's detachment from parents.

Hardgrove and Dawson (1972) claim that contentions concerning children's upset in the presence of parents are based on a number of questionable assumptions. The argument assumes that all display of emotion by children in the presence of parents is undesirable, rather than a positive sign as Robertson suggests. Secondly, the argument assumes that the children are content and happy except when in the presence of their parents, an assumption certainly negated by observation. Hardgrove and Dawson note, however, that a staff member, predisposed to the belief that parents cause upset in children will be able to find evidence of it:

> A crying child alone . . . is seen by the nurse as simply a crying child, a natural enough phenomenon in the hospital. A crying child whose mother has just arrived, however, is seen as a child whose mother is upsetting him unnecessarily by her presence and who would probably be happier if she were not there (p. 8).

Myth 2: Visitation Causes Cross Infection

Opponents of liberal visitation may further argue the dangers of cross infection inherent in such a policy change. From a standpoint of infection control, highly restricted visitation was crucial in the first half of the 20th Century. Infections would sweep through pediatric units, raising the mortality rates to alarming levels. In more recent years the ability to control infection has improved so greatly that restrictive visitation is no longer justifiable on these grounds. As long ago as 1949 some hospitals removed restrictions on visitation, reasoning that the risk of infection was minor as compared to the hazards of separation (Jacoby, 1969). Several studies since that time have confirmed the belief that visitation does not markedly increase the dangers of cross infection (Pickerill and Pickerill, 1954; Lowbury and Jackson, 1960; Barnett et al., 1970; Umphenour, 1980). When questioned whether the very liberal visitation policies at his hospital increased the risk of cross infection, Dr. Marvin Ack, administrator at the Minneapolis Children's Health Center, replied "Nonsense. Doctors are probably more responsible for infection than visitors (Marano and Daniel, 1978)."

Myth 3: Rooming-In Requires Special Facilities

In some settings hospital personnel may agree that parental rooming-in and open visitation are excellent ideas, although they are unworkable in their particular facility. Hardgrove and Dawson (1972) caution against persuasion by such arguments. Rather than waiting for promises of future accommodations for parents which may never materialize, presently existing conditions should be adapted for use by families. A parent who wants to stay with an ill child will make do with a mat on the floor next to the child's bed.

Myth 4: Liberalized Visitation Produces Chaos

A number of other objections to the removal of restrictions on visitation arise from the fears of staff members that chaos and catastrophe will result from "throwing the doors open." Reluctant personnel visualize hoards of parents roaming the unit, dangerously overcrowding important work areas, behaving inappropriately, and demanding services from an already overworked staff. Trouble with large numbers of healthy and highly ambulatory siblings is also anticipated. Such worries cannot be ignored, for such problems may arise if not planned for. Opponents of liberal visitation may seize on such conditions as evidence that the new policies were misguided and deserve to be revoked. To avoid such retrenchment an initial period of planning must occur. The section which follows will deal with important considerations in planning services for parents.

PLANNING FOR PARENTAL ROOMING-IN

The nature of a rooming-in program in a given hospital will be determined in large part by the architecture of the facility, the needs of the patients, and the desires of the staff. Hardgrove and Dawson (1972) provide an excellent review of the types of programs instituted in various settings, and of the problems encountered and overcome in establishing them.

Approaches to Rooming-In

The programs discussed by Hardgrove and Dawson fit into two basic categories: care-by-parent units and rooming-in on the pediatric unit.

Care by Parent Units

A limited number of hospitals (among them, Henrietta Egleston Hospital for Children in Atlanta, Georgia; the University of Kentucky Medical Center in Lexington; James Whitcomb Riley Hospital for Children in Indianapolis; and Boston Floating Hospital) have established special units to which parents are admitted with their children. In such units parents live with their children and retain the role of primary caregiver. Supervisory nurses train parents in the skills they will utilize, such as taking and recording vital signs, measuring urine out-put, monitoring IV's, and giving medications. The costs incurred by the family on care-by-parent units are generally less than that in a normal pediatric ward, because a smaller nursing staff is required, but more important than the financial benefits are the emotional gains for parent and child. Rather than being usurped by hospital personnel, the role of the parent is enhanced in such a setting. The added responsibilities given these parents helps them feel that they are indeed necessary to the care of their children. This knowledge, plus the renewed confidence it generates, makes parents feel more relaxed in the hospital environment, and consequently better able to help the children.

In some hospitals preexisting facilities have been converted to a care-by-parent unit through remodelling, and others have been included in plans for the construction of a new facility.

Rooming-In on the Pediatric Unit

More common than care-by-parent units are facilities which permit rooming-in of parents on the regular pediatric unit. Some more modern facilities were built with parents in mind, providing extra sleep area in the patients' rooms, parent lounges, and shower facilities. Others, recognizing the importance of parents, have attempted to adapt older units, despite their inadequacies. The degree of parental participation in such units varies greatly, depending upon the philosophy of the institution and the attitude of the staff. In some settings, parents are merely visitors, while in others they are truly integrated into the care of their children.

Establishing Procedures and Guidelines

Once the policy of rooming-in has been established and a basic format selected, the focus of efforts must shift from "How do we get parents in here?" to "What do we do with parents once they are here?" A certain amount of planning must take place to insure its benefit to the family and to retain the approval of hospital personnel. Physical arrangements must be considered. Sleeping accommodations for parents must be provided. If at all possible parents should be permitted to sleep in the same room with their child. If space limitations preclude this in certain settings or rooms, a near-by room, perhaps the playroom, can be converted to a dormitory for nighttime hours. Parents should be provided with something to sleep on such as a mat or a fold-up cot. Lounge chairs or chair-beds are more comfortable, but where space is limited and funds scarce, they may be impractical.

Personal areas should also be available to parents. Shower facilities and storage areas are necessary, especially for parents from out of town or on a prolonged stay. Failure to provide such facilities transmits a message to parents that they are not really welcome. Food service must also be available to all rooming-in parents.

The hours in the hospital can grow long and tedious for undiverted parents. They should have access to a parent lounge area where people can gather to relax over coffee with other parents, read, or catch up on work that may be neglected during the period of a child's hospitalization.

When formulating guidelines for a new program, the temptation often exists to consider and provide for every eventuality. To do so, however, may make the program overly restrictive and actually discourage parents from participating. Rules may so narrowly define what a parent may do while with a hospitalized child that the benefit gained from the presence of parents is all but eliminated. For example, a number of hospitals which permit rooming-in deny children access to their parents during the most critical, stressful events, i.e. during blood tests and treatments, during induction of anesthesia, in the recovery room, etc. Reporting results of her survey of hospitals which permit rooming-in of parents, Hardgrove (1980) is critical of the apparent contradiction between liberalized visitation and restrictive policies that separate children from their parents when they are most needed for emotional support:

> Lack of understanding about the reason for parent inclusion may lead to certain counter-productive practices. For example, 77 percent of the respondents asked nothing more of parents than that they offer psychological support and parenting activities to their children, but restricted parents from offering such support during the most stressful times when the child's need for parental reassurance was greatest. Twenty-nine percent do not allow parents to be present during tests and procedures; 89 percent do not allow parents to be with a child during induction of anesthesia; and 81 percent restrict parents from the recovery room (p. 222).

Such misguided over-regulation, ironically even in institutions that permit rooming-in, robs the child of support at times when it is most needed.

Personnel formulating guidelines should restrict their efforts to those areas where potentially major problems are anticipated. Those responsible for transmitting full and accurate information to parents should be designated, so that parents are not subjected to differing stories from several sources concerning the condition of their child. Services provided by the various disciplines should be clarified so that no one feels that he or she is being unfairly over-burdened by the sudden increased presence of parents. Appropriate areas for parent lounges and showers should be determined to avoid conflicts over use of rooms necessary for patient care.

Much of the rooming-in plan should evolve over time, with the suggestions and consultation of the parents being an important part of the developmental process. Through the actual operation of the program, weaknesses can be observed and remedied. Ideas for the improvement or addition of certain elements of the rooming-in program will begin to emerge as parents and staff grow more comfortable in one another's presence.

Problems of day to day operation and management of rooming-in can easily be dealt with if a forum for addressing these concerns exists. A daily meeting for all parents who are rooming-in, such as that held at San Francisco's Moffitt Hospital, provides an excellent opportunity for parents to gather with staff to learn particulars on rooming-in, to voice concerns, and to make basic decisions (Hardgrove and Rutledge, 1975). On the daily agenda is the setting of priorities for the limited bed spaces available for parents. According to the authors, "Preference is given to the parents whose child is in a medical crisis demanding their presence; or is five years old or younger; or is anxious and upset and needs the parents' comfort during the first one or two nights of his stay (p. 837)." Those parents who wish to stay but are not alloted a bed during the meeting are not discouraged from staying, but are advised to bring their own sleeping bags or cots to the hospital.

Prior consideration of the major problems inherent in a rooming-in program and judicious restraint in the formulation of guidelines will allow the new program to gain a fortuitous start. Careful monitoring and sympathetic attention to the concerns and suggestions of parents can assure successful continuation.

INFORMATION AND SUPPORT NEEDED BY ALL PARENTS

Parents typically enter the hospital at less than the peak of their capacities. Concern over the welfare of their children mingles with anxieties fostered by the peculiarities of the hospital setting. Inability to voice complaints is common among an adult population conditioned to accept passively the authority of medical personnel. It is naive to believe that merely because services to parents are part of official hospital policy they will be readily and effectively utilized. Parents mired in the stress of a child's hospitalization need an ally among the hospital staff who can provide information concerning available services and give emotional support to the parents so they, in turn, are better able to help their children.

Ideally, a full-time position of parent advocate or parent coordinator should be created and charged with the duties of safeguarding parents' rights and actively dispensing services to parents. Too often, however, these important duties are delegated to, or divided among, other existing disciplines, including social work, nursing, and child life. Whether the child life worker assumes primary responsibility for implementation of parent programs, or merely works in close cooperation with those who do, he or she must be fully aware of the needs of parents who must admit a child for hospitalization.

Of paramount importance to parents is their need for full and accurate information. Much of the discomfort experienced by parents in the hospital environment arises from their lack of knowledge in a variety of areas. In addition to the basic information on the condition of their children, parents also need to know about such seemingly trivial matters as what they should bring to the hospital or where they-should stand during an examination of their child. While such information may seem mundane, it serves to reassure the parents, thereby making them feel more welcome and relaxed. The power of increasing information to parents was dramatically demonstrated by Skipper and Leonard (1968), in the study discussed in the previous chapter. Their research showed that the children of parents who received a greater degree of information than was normal for the hospital studied showed less physiological stress, recuperated more rapidly, and demonstrated less post-hospital upset than children whose parents received the usual amount of information.

Conveying Information Before Admission

The flow of information to parents must not wait until the child is admitted. By that time a number of common questions will have undoubtedly arisen. If they are answered immediately, the parent receives a relaxing reassurance; if unanswered, the questions may produce needless anxiety. In the case related at the beginning of this chapter, Mrs. Johnson's lack of knowledge concerning appropriate means of preparing Heather forced her to act upon well-meaning, but misguided, instinct. Mrs. Johnson's fear that she had failed Heather created a sense of guilt and anxiety, easily detected by the child, amplifying her own fears.

Two principal mechanisms exist through which the child life worker and other interested health care professionals can transmit essential information to parents and children prior to the day of admission: a preadmission preparation booklet and a preadmission familiarization program or hospital tour.

Preadmission Preparation Booklet

The preadmission booklet can be mailed directly to the family, or special arrangements can be made with physicians to have it dispensed from their offices. The material contained in this booklet should be simply and clearly stated, allowing for parents who have poor reading skills, and should cover those topics of greatest concern to parents. Hardgrove (undated) has compiled a list of subject areas about which parents need information. These topics, which should be included in the preadmission booklet, are as follows:

(1) What to tell their child

(2) What to wear and what to bring

(3) Whom to turn to (and when) for accurate information and for support

(4) How to behave on the unit

(5) How to help one's child (parenting care plans)

(6) What are parents expected to do? What are they allowed to do?

WHAT TO TELL THEIR CHILD. Many parents are unaware of the extreme necessity of preparing their children for the experience of hospitalization. The preadmission booklet should urge parents to talk with their children about the upcoming event, providing guidelines for this activity. A coloring book or story about the hospital serves as an excellent vehicle for facilitating the parent-child discussions, introducing the types of equipment, people, and routines the child will encounter. The coloring-/story-book can be part of the preadmission booklet or an appropriate children's book available in the local library can be recommended. Further instructions for a basic explanation of the child's specific reason for hospitalization may supplement the booklet, as may suggestions for appropriate play activities.

The booklet should also tell parents of the availability of rooming-in facilities, so that from the earliest moments of preparation the child can be aware that a parent will stay with him or her at the hospital.

WHAT TO WEAR AND WHAT TO BRING. Parents need to know how to pack for their children, and for themselves, should they choose to exercise their rooming-in privilege. If children will be provided with pajamas and toothbrushes, parents should be made aware of this. The desirability and permissibleness of having a child bring a favorite toy from home (properly marked, to avoid losing it in the playroom!) should also be explained. The importance of the child's having street clothes to wear when he or she can get out of bed might also be emphasized.

Those parents who plan to room-in should be given a realistic picture of the availability of storage space, so they can plan their wardrobe accordingly. Other information, such as the availability of laundry facilities or the proximity of stores, should be provided.

WHOM TO TURN TO. As Skipper and Leonard (1968) observed, "the hospital is a notoriously poor organization for eliciting information, for providing support, or generating a reassuring atmosphere (p. 275)." To avoid undue frustration and anxiety, parents should be aware of all sources of information and support they will find in the hospital. Appropriate sources of medical information should be identified, and the roles of other supportive personnel clarified. The identification of parent advocate, child life worker, social worker or other professional responsible for coordinating parent services should, of course, receive prominent attention. Parents should also know the time and place for regularly scheduled parent meetings, if any exist.

How to Behave on the Unit. Much of what the staff may perceive to be insensitive behavior on the part of parents may actually be the result of parents acting out of ignorance. Hardgrove (undated) notes instances in which parents leave the hospital when their presence is most desireable to the staff and their children, i.e. at meal time or during treatments. Parents may watch TV or gather for chats at times when children should be in bed. Tension and conflict that could potentially arise from such situations can be avoided if parents are aware of a few basic guidelines and are familiar with the pediatric unit's schedule.

How to Help One's Child. In traditional health care settings parents are often made to feel useless and unimportant to their children. They yield their ill child to the medical staff upon admission and adopt the role of passive, helpless observers of the child's care, afraid to even touch their child unless granted permission by hospital personnel. Information contained in the preadmission booklet should dispel this image, assuring parents of their importance, and offering simple suggestions of how they may be helpful to their child before and during the hospitalization.

What are Parents Expected to do: Obviously, any special expectations of the parents must be fully clarified. For example, in care-by-parent settings parents must be aware of the types of functions they may be called upon to perform. Information concerning other important preadmission activities, such as the hospital tour, laboratory tests, or preoperative physical examinations, should be included.

Parents should also be told exactly what types of activities are permissible while in the hospital. Parents intimidated by the hospital environment may assume that anesthesia induction facilities and the recovery room are forbidden territories unless informed otherwise, and thus deny their children crucial support through their absence.

Ideally, of course, the preadmission booklet should be written by hospital personnel so that it contains specific information about that particular hospital. If for some reason that is not possible, a more general booklet, purchased from an outside source, might be considered. Perhaps the best choice is *When Your Child Goes to the Hospital*, available for 85 cents from the Superintendent of Documents, Government Printing Office, Washington, D.C. 20402 (stock # 017-091-00217-7).

Preadmission Orientation Program

As important and comprehensive as the information in the preadmission booklet may be, it should never be allowed to serve as the sole source of information prior to hospitalization. Parents may fail to read the material carefully, either because of their own limited reading skills, time constraints, or their own anxieties and wishes to deny the reality of the impending event. All of this information should be repeated when parents bring their children to the hospital for a preadmission familiarization tour. Although the oral presentation of this material is primarily important for those parents who had not previously read it, it serves a useful function for all. The fact that a sympathetic, understanding member of the hospital staff (the child life worker or someone else) has taken time to inform and reassure parents symbolizes a desire by the hospital to provide humane, comprehensive care. Rather than remaining frozen in print, hospital policy comes alive and pursues the cooperation of parents. The oral presentation format further allows parents to ask questions and clarify matters, a practice which should be encouraged as they prepare to enter the hospital setting.

Naturally, parents who have neglected to read preadmission information, or who are hampered by their own fears of hospitals, cannot be expected to take advantage of a preadmission tour and orientation unless the hospital staff makes special efforts to invite them in addition to mailing an announcement. A call by the child life worker, encouraging the family to come to the preadmission orientation and explaining the importance of such a visit prior to hospitalization is an effective way of increasing participation in this program.

Conveying Information After Admission

Once parents and child have entered the hospital, the flow of information concerning the condition of the child, hospital routines, and available parent services should continue through a variety of media. Regularly scheduled parent meetings are an excellent vehicle through which a member of the nursing staff can communicate with parents and answer their questions. Hardgrove and Dawson (1972) suggest the use of parent bulletin boards, wall signs, and maps depicting the pediatric unit and other important hospital areas. Coffee breaks can be instituted, during which parents can gather informally with representatives of various hospital disciplines that are in less frequent contact with parents. For example, someone from the business office might be available to answer general questions about health insurance and hospital costs, or an administrator might discuss hospital philosophy and goals.

The information generally of most concern to parents is the medical condition of their child. A number of basic questions concerning routines and procedures can be answered as parents participate in the child's preparation by the child life worker, thereby reassuring and benefitting both parents and child. As the work of Wolfer and Visintainer (1975) reveals, preparation of parents and their children together results in lowered parental anxiety and increased satisfaction with nursing care, while improving the child's adjustment in the hospital and upon discharge. For more detailed information on the content of preparation sessions, see Chapter 6.

Dispensing information specific to the current medical condition of the child lies outside the immediate province of child life workers, although they can support the parents' probing for information in several ways. First, child life workers can continually remind their colleagues of parents' need for open communication and a constant up-dating of information. Second, particular instances of concern expressed by parents can be reported by child life workers to the appropriate parties. Finally, the child life worker who senses that a parent is reluctant to ask questions of nurses or physicians due to fear or intimidation should offer support and encouragement to enable the parent to approach those figures directly.

Questions of a nonmedical nature, particularly those concerning parenting skills or child development issues, should be handled by the child life worker. If the demand seems great enough, the child life staff can develop programs and materials covering topics of interest to parents and families.

Providing Support for Parents

As is obvious from the preceding discussion, information alone, though reassuring to parents, is insufficient to see them through the hospital experience. A study by Gofman et al. (1957) found that 57 percent of the parents whose children were hospitalized experienced "overwhelming" anxiety. While an aggressive and thorough program of information transmission will undoubtedly improve this condition, all parents will still require some degree of support. For some parents, that emotional support which is an integral part of the previously described programs will be sufficient. They will feel welcome and comfortable in the hospital environment and will find that the concerned efforts of hospital personnel permit them to function admirably, despite the stresses of the situation.

Other parents, however, require more intensive efforts. It is quite common for parents to experience guilt over the admission of a child to the hospital, feeling that their increased vigilence could have detected illness at an earlier, less serious stage, or that greater attention to safety could have prevented a child's accident. The financial burdens of an extended hospitalization may weigh heavily on the minds of parents. If, in dealing with parents, child life workers find parents to be immobilized by these or other concerns, and that their efforts to help the parents cope with such feelings are ineffective, other sources of support must be sought. Personnel in the departments of social work, psychology, and psychiatry will prove to be valuable allies in the child life worker's attempt to ease the strain of hospitalization for parents.

Guidelines for Supportive Listening

Even though referral to mental health professionals in another department may be helpful in serious cases of parental stress, it is neither possible nor desirable to refer to a counselor every parent who has concerns to express. At random times and in a variety of settings, parents may begin to talk to the child life worker about feelings or problems related to the child's hospitalization. Since the child life worker is not directly involved in the medical treatment of the child, parents often feel more inclined to discuss their problems with a child life worker than with a physician or nurse. On these occasions, it is helpful if the child life worker knows how to listen supportively to parents. While they can never replace a course in helping or counseling skills, the guidelines below offer specific suggestions for listening to parents:

(1) Keep the focus of the conversation on the parent. Don't steal the spotlight by talking about your own experiences, giving advice, making interpretations, or offering suggestions. Keep the speaker in center stage.

(2) Look directly at the speaker.

(3) Nod your head and say "uh-huh" or "umm-humm" from time to time to signal that you are paying attention.

(4) Don't be afraid of silence. When the parent pauses, resist the impulse to fill the silence with chatter. The parent will probably continue talking when it's apparent that you're willing to continue listening.

(5) Draw out the parent with questions. Use open-ended questions to encourage the speaker to talk some more: "How did you feel about that?" "Can you tell me more about that?" Avoid questions that can be answered "yes" or "no" or with a simple one-word answer.

(6) If you disagree with what the parent is saying, avoid using questions to lead him or her to see things your way. "Leading" questions discourage the parent rather than indicating that you wish to hear that person's point of view.

(7) Use perception checks (restating what you have heard) to make sure you are understanding accurately what the speaker is saying. When it is clear the parent has finished one aspect of the discussion,

paraphrase or summarize the main idea expressed, asking the parent to correct you if you have misunderstood. A perception check often starts with a phrase such as, "Then you're saying that you . . ." or "It seems that you're saying . . ." or "You think . . . . is that right?"

(8) Respond to feeling messages. Show that you understand how the parent is feeling as well as what he or she is saying. Such statements might begin, "You must be feeling pretty angry about that . . ." or "I guess you're feeling pretty . . ."

In addition to listening supportively to the parents' concerns, the child life worker can offer support to parents by helping them deal with the practical problems engendered by having a child in the hospital. If transportation to the hospital is a problem for parents, possible solutions can be explored by the child life worker or other staff members. Special arrangements with bus or cab companies might be made, or a listing of volunteer drivers compiled. For those parents who have difficulty leaving home because of the presence of other children, the hospital might create a sibling play area under child life supervision, or the volunteer department might develop a program for providing homemaking services. Other problems should be similarly addressed to insure the maximum participation of parents in the care of their hospitalized children.

Providing Parents with a Role

The ultimate goal of efforts to invite parents into the pediatric facility and to encourage their participation in the care of the child is to preserve the parent-child relationship from which the child can derive so much essential strength. Parents must be continually reminded through the actions and encouragement of all hospital staff that the child, though hospitalized, remains *their* child. While parents may be comfortable with their role outside the hospital, the role of "parent in hospital" is new and perhaps threatening. By suggesting specific tasks for parents, e.g. taking vital signs, feeding their children, and monitoring IV's, and providing certain expectations (staying with a child during induction of anesthesia, being present in the recovery room, staying overnight) the hospital helps parents become more comfortable in the new role.

The child life worker, whose principal contacts with parents will be in conjunction with preparation and play activities, must be aware of the discomfort and insecurities parents may feel as they attempt to become "parents in the hospital." The temptation may exist for the child life worker to focus too narrowly on the child in the presence of parents. If parents are present for either a preparation or play session, they should be encouraged to participate fully. The child life worker should scrupulously avoid usurping the parents' role as provider of play. Instead, the child life worker can supplement and enhance that role, by teaching parents new ways of playing with their children and serving as a role model for parents who may feel uncomfortable with play activities. By helping parents to play better with their children, the child life worker is imparting an important skill which will follow the family home from the hospital.

Not all play can, or necessarily should, take place in the presence of parents. Parents much in need of a period of time away from their child may welcome the arrival of the child life worker for a play session. If parents need to leave the hospital, they should do so with the assurance of the child life worker that the child will be able to play busily during their absence. At other times the child life worker may wish to schedule a play session alone with the child, especially if it seems that the child's play is inhibited by parents, or if the child seems to have concerns centering around the parents which might be disclosed in play. Even at these times, the child life worker should be cognizant of the needs and feelings of parents so as to avoid undue usurpation of a role which is rightfully theirs.

The Child Life Worker and Siblings

The presence of siblings in the hospital as a means of supporting the hospitalized child, monitoring their adaptation to the hospitalized child's illness, and maintaining the family unit, has been previously discussed. The child life worker can facilitate the inclusion of non-hospitalized siblings in hospital activities in several ways. Siblings can be included in the play of the hospitalized children, with the assistance and encouragement of the child life staff. For those children on bedrest, a brother or sister can assure a constant source of play. Ambulatory patients can bring their siblings to the playroom for group activities and special events.

A sibling play area, supervised by child life personnel, can provide a place for children to play when a brother or sister is too ill to visit, when the hospitalized sibling is undergoing surgery or another procedure, or if the hospitalized child is considerably older or younger. Siblings feel proud and pleased to have their own special place at the hospital where they can explore and play as they attempt to deal with their feelings about this strange new environment. The trained and watchful child life worker is present to guide them in this pursuit.

Summary

The event of hospitalization places severe strains on the fabric of family life. If the family is unsupported during this critical time, the stress may contribute to family disintegration or provoke psychological distress among its individual members. Concerned hospital personnel must work to maintain family relationships in the transition from home to hospital and back. Through aggressive and thorough dissemination of information, appropriate support, and extreme sensitivity to the needs of all family members, the child life worker and other concerned health care professionals can minimize the disruption caused by the hospitalization of a child.

(For further guidance in working with parents and families, see Appendix B.)

CHAPTER 4

THE IMPORTANCE OF PLAY
TO THE HOSPITALIZED CHILD

THE GREEN HULK PLAYS DOCTOR

"The Green Hulk" trudged his way toward the playroom, with shoulders hunched forward and glistening teeth bared. A pair of young toddlers scurried as "the Hulk" kicked toys and blocks from his path. Geoff, the child life worker on duty in the playroom, studied the creature's movements from the table where he and several children had been exploring the mysterious properties of magnets. Earlier that evening Geoff had met five-year-old Josh, well before Josh's transformation into his current monster-like state. Geoff recalled that Josh was admitted for a hernia repair, which was to be performed the next morning. A quick recollection of the conversation he had held with Josh's mother reminded Geoff that Josh would be spending the night alone.

"Hi, Josh! Would you like to join us?" Geoff inquired, with a motion toward the magnets scattered across the table.

"I'm not Josh. I'm 'the Hulk,'" corrected Josh.

Excusing himself from the table, Geoff approached the monster. "Boy, you look pretty angry, Hulk! What's going on?"

A growl was the only reply.

Realizing that Josh was not ready to yield any recognizable verbal clues identifying the source of his anger, Geoff tried a different approach. The Hulk interrupted his rampage to watch as Geoff assembled a yard-high tower from wooden blocks. Grabbing a bean bag from the shelf, Geoff sent it sailing toward the tower, demolishing it in an instant!

The Hulk emitted a growl of delight and jumped around in a circle.

"Have you ever tried this before, Hulk?"

Without a word of response, Josh lunged toward the blocks and resurrected the structure. Once again the bean bag worked its destruction, encouraged by the increasingly gleeful growls. As Josh alternately built and demolished the tower, Geoff observed the gradual dissipation of Josh's tension.

Although pleased that Josh had been able to discharge some of his anger through the vigorous throwing of the bean bag, Geoff felt it important that Josh explore a variety of play materials. By so doing, Josh might "play through" situations or conditions that were troubling

60

him, perhaps revealing their nature to the child life worker.

Geoff directed Josh to a corner of the playroom that contained medical play equipment, including many authentic hospital instruments, as well as puppets, a doll family, and dress-up clothing.

Josh eagerly examined the materials, pausing occasionally to concentrate on specific items. The doll family and a needle-less syringe were of particular interest to him. Geoff watched as Josh repeatedly gave injections to the girl doll of the family.

"Well, Dr. Josh, how is your patient?" Geoff inquired.

"Real bad. Her heart stopped beating."

"Will you be able to help her, Doctor?"

"Uh, I think so. This shot will do it," reported the young physician.

"How does your patient feel, Dr. Josh?"

"She's all better now," Josh replied. Tossing the doll back among the others, Josh took a seat at the table with the other children, where he played contentedly with the magnets until it was time for bed.

Geoff was uncertain of the significance of this play, or of the circumstances that precipitated Josh's initial anger. Perhaps Josh had some concerns that hadn't been fully revealed during his preparation session. Josh may have been angry at his parents for leaving him alone at the hospital. He may have been jealous of a sister who was allowed to remain at home. Whatever it all meant, Geoff was relieved to see that the play had a calming effect on the child and seemingly helped him resolve some undisclosed conflict.

After seeing the children off to their rooms for the night, Geoff recorded his observations of Josh's play in the young patient's chart, alerting other health care professionals to watch for possible difficulties being experienced by Josh.

UNDERSTANDING JOSH'S PLAY

The anger and anxiety manifested by Josh's rampage in the form of the Hulk is not unusual. Anyone, be it adult or child, will experience feelings of discomfort, hostility or rage when suddenly thrust into the hospital and confronted with its numerous peculiarities. People often bristle at the regimentation and passivity required of the patient role, or resent frequent invasions of privacy. Such feelings, if secretly harbored by the discontented patient, can produce or aggravate other problems which potentially interfere with the patient's recovery. For example, a patient who is angered by the insensitive manner of a physician, but unable to express that anger, may react indirectly through uncooperative behavior and distrust of the staff as a whole. To avoid such counterproductive occurrences, the hospital staff should continually encourage expression of patients' feelings about hospitalization. With adolescents and adults, verbal interaction is the vehicle for meeting this goal, although most hospitals are admittedly inadequate in facilitating the ventilation of feelings.

Verbal disclosure of feelings is often more difficult for young patients than for their older counterparts. The language of many, particularly preschoolers, is not highly developed, impeding the accurate assignment of words to the frequently subtle shades of feelings. Also, the scary nature of a child's thoughts may make him or her reluctant to express them, even if the verbal capacity to do so exists. Children who feel hatred of their parents for bringing them to the hospital or contempt for the medical staff for inflicting pain may avoid revealing these feelings for fear of retribution from such powerful figures.

Despite the problems inherent in verbal communication, the child may still allow us to monitor changing moods or discover the nature of gnawing concerns through observation of the child's play. Our friend Josh was upset for some reason which he wouldn't readily disclose to the child life worker. His adopted mode of play, transformation into the character of the Green Hulk, communicated his anger to those around him. Josh was fortunate that his play was seen by a sensitive, understanding person who knew how to encourage his play and enable him to deal with his concerns more effectively. In another hospital, less cognizant of the necessity of play for its patients, Josh might have been denied this opportunity. If no playroom existed, he might have been forced to confine his anger to his room, perhaps becoming destructive. He may have internalized his anger, becoming depressed and withdrawing from the medical staff, a condition which certainly could have retarded his recovery. Had Josh, for lack of proper play facilities, taken the Hulk to a hectic nurses' station, he might have incurred the wrath of the staff and been considered a "behavior problem." The presence of a skilled child life worker enabled Josh to express and confront his feelings in an appropriate manner, decreasing, rather than compounding, the difficulties of hospitalization.

Play facilitates the child's self-expression and provides a mechanism for coping with difficulties. Play allows a child to become an active participant, rather than the passive receiver so often the norm in a hospital experience. While in the playroom Josh was able to be a vigorous actor, throwing the bean bag, handling the syringe, and manipulating the dolls and other play equipment in any manner he desired. He was permitted to regain a feeling of power denied him in other spheres of the hospital.

As well as promoting the emotional health of the hospitalized child, play is important to the child's normal development. The negative effects of hospitalization on development can be minimized through a thorough and thoughtful program of play. From observing Josh's behavior in the playroom, one can easily see how the so-called therapeutic aspects of play (concentrating on the emotional adjustment of the child to the hospital setting) intertwine with the other forms of developmental play. For example, the building and toppling of the block tower was an excellent way to discharge anger, but it also afforded practice in the physical skills of balancing objects and throwing accurately. Further opportunity to practice fine motor manipulations arose as Josh learned to handle the syringe and as he explored the magnets.

The playroom setting also provided intellectual stimulation necessary to promote learning while a child is hospitalized. While playing with the syringe, Josh might have noticed that air rushes out the top when the plunger is depressed, or that the plunger is hard to depress when the tip is firmly covered with a finger. Josh undoubtedly learned a great deal as he maneuvered the magnets to repel or attract each other.

These emotional, physical, and intellectual activities occurred in the presence of other people, including children of Josh's age. Thus Josh was permitted to explore social development through the course of his play. He was likely aware of the reaction of others to his various forms of play. When he decided that it was time to play with others at the table, it was necessary for Josh to call upon and practice social skills such as peer communication and cooperation. If group play were not encouraged, Josh and other children would be denied this important experience.

The various forms of play in which hospitalized children engage and their special importance during this stressful period will be discussed in this chapter. By better understanding the beneficial effects of play in coping with the stress and anxiety related to hospitalization and main taining normal growth and development, the child life worker can more effectively meet the needs of the hospitalized child.

THE NECESSITY FOR PLAY

When considering the possibility of establishing a child life program at her facility, one director of nursing remarked, "I don't think the administrator would ever allow us to hire a full-time person *just to play with the kids.*" This type of thinking is sadly prevalent among hospital personnel and represents a severe misunderstanding of the essential role of play in the life of the child. Most adults reflect fondly upon the carefree play of their earlier years, recalling messes made, dangers encountered, secret clubs, and make-believe. The same adults take a cursory look at the play of children today and find a similar characteristic glee and spontaneity. Play is, to be sure, a wonderously pleasurable activity, but to concentrate only on this element of play is to miss its true significance. Too many people, the above-mentioned director of nursing included, tend to equate play with frivolity, viewing it as a nice diversion for children but not something to be taken seriously. Thus, hospital play programs may be seen as a nice frill, such as in-room television or a gift shop, rather than an essential part of the child's care.

Scholars have described play in various ways in an attempt to convey a feeling of its importance in the life of a child. Play has been called the work of childhood, a description which emphasizes the seriousness of the activity by comparing it to an adult occupation. Others have called play the child's response to life, underscoring the inextricable link between the play of children and the world around them. Hartley and Goldenson (1963) have modified this description, noting that "play is not only the child's response to life; it *is* his life, if he is to be a vital, growing,creative individual (p. 1)."

Children deprived of adequate opportunities to play and explore may experience difficulties in various aspects of their development. The failure of some infants to gain weight and thrive in a normal manner has in many cases been attributed to insufficient stimulation or human interaction. Such infants show marked improvement when an organized program of play and interaction is initiated.

Intellectual development of the child may also be impeded by paucity of play experiences. A study quoted by Knight (1978) indicated that "children under five years of age who live above the third floor of an apartment dwelling have limited access to play space and play opportunities. They don't go down to play as often and when they do they don't play out as long (p. 48)." As a result, the study revealed, children who lived above the ninth floor (and who were, therefore, less able to take advantage of the normal play experiences available at street level) were, on the average, almost one year behind those children on lower floors in terms of intellectual growth.

A number of authors have discussed the emotional, physical, and intellectual problems which classically occurred among institutionalized children. Casler (1961) has attributed much of this problem to the lack of stimulation characterizing such environments. If materials were available to the children and social encouragement provided, institutionalized children would more readily and actively explore and interact with their environment, minimizing the disastrous effects of such a situation.

Since play is such an integral part of the life of children, and since its suppression can so severely handicap normal growth and development, children in the hospital, even for a brief duration, should have ample opportunity to engage in this activity. The child's urge to play is so strong that even when denied proper space and materials, he or she will utilize whatever is available, be it ashtrays, IV poles, or light switches, in order to continue. Rather than frustrating the child's insatiable urge to play, forcing him or her to seek less desirable or even dangerous play media like these, the hospital should facilitate it through the activities of the child life program.

WHAT IS PLAY?

We have all engaged in it and readily recognize it when we see it; yet the formulation of a definition of play is difficult. Mark Twain once commented on the paradoxical nature of play, noting that a person who fashions an artificial flower for pay is "working" while another who undertakes a vigorous mountain climb is said to be at play. The latter of these activities requires great concentration, physical exhaustion, and, perhaps, even pain; yet the person performing this activity freely choses to do so, and, presumably, derives pleasure from the pursuit. This would seem to be play. The flower maker, on the other hand, is engaged in this activity with a predetermined goal of earning money, rather than spontaneously enjoying a pleasurable pastime. Most people would agree with Twain that such an activity is not play. Yet when we observe a child in a hospital playroom making a flower from pipe-cleaners and tissue paper, we feel confident saying that this is a child at play!

Garvey (1977) has compiled a list of elements which characterize play. A review of these characteristics will help to clarify the reasons for considering some activities play, while excluding others of a very similar nature:

(1) Play is pleasurable, enjoyable. Even when not actually accompanied by signs of mirth, it is still positively valued by the player.

(2) Play has no extrinsic goals. Its motivations are intrinsic and serve no other objectives. In fact, it is more an enjoyment of means than an effort devoted to some particular end. In utilitarian terms, it is inherently unproductive.

(3) Play is spontaneous and voluntary. It is not obligatory but is freely chosen by the player.

(4) Play involves some active engagement on the part of the player.

(5) Play has certain systematic relations to what is not play (p. 4–5).

Play Is Pleasurable

The pleasurable aspect of play is often readily observable. One need only walk through the pediatric ward of a hospital committed to play to find evidence of this fact. In one room an infant slaps a musical mobile and giggles in response, while her roommate plays a gleeful game of "peek-a-boo" with his mother. A group of preschoolers in the playroom proudly skip and march to the beat of a volunteer play leader's tom-tom. Outside the playroom two school-age males compare techniques in the handling of their wheelchairs, each laughing as the other demonstrates his prowess. The smiles and laughter of these children convey their feelings of enjoyment.

Even in the absence of these obvious indicators of amusement, the child derives pleasure from play. A four-year-old boy stands at the playroom sink, vigorously scouring a small pile of play dishes. Pausing for a brief inspection, he notices a stubborn spot and returns to his scrubbing. At a table a few feet away, a seven-year-old girl puts the finishing touches on a bridge she has constructed from plastic blocks. Her face reflects the concern of an engineer seeking to insure the safety of future passengers over the structure. Despite a façade of seriousness, both children are highly engrossed in their pursuits, gaining a sense of pleasure from their freely chosen activities.

Play Has No Extrinsic Goals

The child engages in play for its own sake, not to gain some other external objective. The flower maker discussed earlier may have derived pleasure from the production of the flower, but this activity is distinguished from the realm of play, since the flower was made with an eye toward the external goal of making money. The four-year-old dishwasher exerted great effort in his activity, yet this child was still involved in a play experience. The process of splashing in the water, holding the suds and squeezing the sponge, in an unconscious parody of adults, was the fun part. Had the child undertaken these actions with the serious goal of cleaning the playroom, the play atmosphere would have evaporated.

Play Is Spontaneous

One cannot be compelled to play. Children choose to play when and where they desire. A sensitive adult can structure potential play experiences for children, with an understanding of a child's interests and needs. Thus, a playroom can be stocked with toys that children are likely to enjoy and can be arranged in a manner conducive to play. But it is the child who accepts or rejects a given invitation to play. A child life worker may, for example, feel that a certain patient would benefit from medical play and therefore may introduce such equipment to the child. A great number of hospitalized children will readily accept an opportunity to handle and operate the equipment that has been used so frequently on them. But others, because of their fears or intimidation, may withdraw. The child life worker may try other approaches or may reintroduce the materials at a later time, but no effort should be made to force the child to participate.

Play Involves Active Engagement

Quite obviously, the child must be actively involved for play to occur. The child who passively sits and watches television (or a magic show in the hospital playroom, for that matter) is not playing. Of the examples of play given previously, most involve energetic physical involvement by the children. Running, marching, building, doing the dishes, or manipulating a wheelchair all demand an active commitment of the child's body to the play experience. That the domain of play requires such an active investment from its participants is especially important in the hospital setting where children are so frequently asked to be very passive. Through play the child can exercise mastery over the environment, even one so foreign as the hospital.

For some hospitalized children physically active participation in the play is difficult. Paralysis, traction, casts, or other impediments may alter the degree to which children can physically engage in play activities, but such conditions in no way diminish the child's desire or need to participate. In fact, the immobilized child may require an increased amount of play. Children should be allowed to engage physically in the play to the limits of their abilities. The child life worker should adapt the activity to suit the condition of the child. In cases in which the child's disabilities are such that he or she is unable to engage physically in a desired activity, the child life worker should serve as a surrogate body, performing manipulations as directed by the child. One nine-year-old boy whose hands were severely burned constructed a marvelously complex structure with glue and popsicle sticks by issuing detailed directives to the child life worker assisting him.

Play Has Systematic Relations to What Is Not Play

The infant batting a mobile is playing, yet in the process is learning to control developing young muscles and to predict cause and effect relationships. The four-year-old dish-washer is, through his play, gaining experience in an adult role. The children moving in step to the drum have freely chosen to enter this pleasurable form of play and, as a consequence, are learning how to function with their peers.

The play of children is characterized by the elements mentioned above. It is a pleasurable active pursuit, freely chosen, with no goal in mind beyond the play itself. In the course of such play, however, children are learning, growing, gaining new skills, and testing new experiences. It is this quality of play that makes it such a superbly effective mechanism as children grow toward adulthood and attempt to cope with the obstacles encountered along the way. Before examining the special significance of play for the hospitalized child, this relationship of play to what is not play will be examined more closely.

THE ROLE OF PLAY IN THE LIFE OF THE CHILD

As children develop physically, intellectually, socially and emotionally, play activities help them discover and test new abilities, perfect these abilities, and advance toward other skills. Any given form of play may, in fact, serve as practice for skills in several areas of development. A simple schoolyard game of tag, for example, challenges a number of the child's developing abilities. Physically, the child must be swift and agile to avoid the tag of a pursuer. Quick stops, starts, and a variety of other body movements must be employed. Intellectually, the child must employ a strategy either to avoid becoming "It" or to transfer that honor to another. In the social realm, the child is learning important group interaction skills. One must approach others to initiate the game, agree upon rules, and arbitrate disputes. Although play generally affects several areas of development at once, it is helpful, for the sake of clarity, to examine each separately.

Play and Physical Development

The physical abilities of newborn infants are minimal. They can neither grasp, sit up, crawl, nor stand; yet in less than a year they will possess all these capabilities and more. Biological maturation permits much of this astounding advancement, as muscles and bones develop to a point sufficient to meet the given task. Yet play provides a large measure of the motivation necessary to exercise the young body and facilitate development. The random motions of an infant's arm may place a hand in contact with an intriguing object such as a rattle. The baby will, over a period of time, make repeated attempts to grasp the rattle or other attractive objects. Eventually the task is accomplished, and additional practice increases the ease with which it is performed. The ability to grasp increases the infant's control of the environment, permitting expanded play opportunities and preparing the way for further developmental advances.

As the child continues to acquire new physical skills, play experiences arise to provide motivation and practice. The child learning to walk plays a game of coming to Mommy or Daddy. Climbing skills are fostered by play on small slides or through expeditions up the stairway. Chase games and imitations of animals provide ample opportunity to practice running, crawling, and jumping.

While large muscle activities such as these are developing, children set about acquiring finer, more sophisticated skills. Here again play accompanies and encourages this development. The child who has learned to grasp a ball begins to practice throwing it. Tireless efforts eventually enable the child to throw the ball with accuracy. Clumsy attempts to grasp a writing implement and make scrawling marks are eventually replaced by recognizable pictures. As the child grows older, artistic techniques, athletics, and other pursuits continue to challenge the child's agility and coordination. Masterful control of extremely fine movements are necessary to thread a needle, for example. To hit a golf ball accurately, strength, plus the coordination of various groups of muscles, must be attained.

The child, of course, does not play in order to develop his or her body, but rather for the pure pleasure inherent in the play. Yet it is through childhood's seemingly insatiable urge to play that new skills, made possible by biological maturation, are discovered and refined.

Play and Intellectual Development

According to Jean Piaget (1970), children learn about the world around them through their own actions and explorations. During the course of their playful experiences, children are continually taking in, or *assimilating*, new information encountered. A young child may have had the opportunity to play with round balloons, noting in the course of the investigation that they have certain properties. They are light in weight, squeezable (but will pop if squeezed too much), have a certain distinctive feel, and, if dropped, will gently float to the ground. When presented with a tubular shaped balloon, the young detective will examine its properties and soon conclude that this too is a balloon. The child has assimilated this new shape into the concept of balloon, but to do so the child had to alter an old way of thinking about balloons—that is, not all balloons are round. The process of altering old patterns of thinking to allow for the further assimilation of information is called *accommodation*.

Our same young detective watches with amazement as an adult produces "balloons" by dipping a looped piece of wire into a thick, glistening liquid and waves the wire through the air. A shower of transparent balloons come floating downward toward the young child, who is anxious to play with them in the accustomed manner. When touched, however, the balloon disappears! The detective searches for clues, but is frustrated in the attempt. There was no pop as there should have been when it burst, nor was there the usual shriveled piece of rubber to be found. Anyway, that light touch shouldn't have popped a balloon. The incredulous child tests another, with similar results. These objects don't fit into the old balloon scheme, so the child makes another accommodation: some round, shiny objects which gently float to the ground are *not* balloons. Soon the child develops new ways of playing with these novel objects, popping them, blowing them higher into the air, and catching them on the cloth of a sleeve.

Through the interaction of assimilation and accommodation intellectual growth occurs, continuing through adulthood. For adults, however, the process may occur on a more abstract plane, with ideas rather than objects being manipulated. The young child, for whom abstract thought is an impossibility, must rely upon direct action in order to assimilate new information and discover the need for accommodation in old patterns. That is, the child must play.

Piaget has described four distinct stages of human intellectual growth, with the play activities of each being characteristically different. (For a more complete review of Piaget's theories, see Flavell [1963].)

Sensorimotor Stage

This stage lasts from birth to about two years of age. During this period children move from the dominance of reflex mechanisms with which they are born, to a deliberate manipulation of objects. Through continual play and observation the child eventually discovers the permanence of objects (that they exist, even when out of the infant's sight) and notices the connection between his or her actions and their effects on objects. Play during this period consists largely of an exploration of a variety of bodily movements and the repetition of those actions which the child finds pleasing.

Preoperational Stage

This period lasts from approximately age two to age seven years. The child who in the previous period developed the concept of object permanence now has a greater ability to hold and recall the image of objects and events, because of the increasing use of symbolization. Mental images and language allow the child to represent objects and relationships in the surrounding world. Children at this age are highly egocentric, incapable of viewing the world from any perspective other than their own.

The play of children during this stage is filled with symbolism. Preoperational children can engage in "pretend" or make-believe play. They imitate objects and recreate events. Play materials may be transformed into a variety of other representations. A set of blocks, for example, may be used to represent buildings, cars, rocks, food, or anything else that the creative young mind wishes.

Concrete Operational Stage

This stage lasts from approximately seven to twelve years of age. Certain mental operations are possible for the child in this period which were beyond the child's capabilities a few years earlier. The concrete operational child has developed a concept of *conservation*, noting that certain properties of liquids and solids (e.g. weight, volume, number of individual items) remain constant despite transformation in length, shape, or grouping. The preoperational child, for example, might say that rolling a ball of clay into a longer shape increases its total mass. The concrete operational child, who now possesses the ability to mentally reverse this operation ("seeing" the clay returned to its original shape) would know that the clay's volume remains constant. Thus, the child of this age is increasingly able to think logically, although such thought processes are, at this point, only possible in the physically concrete realm.

The concrete operational child has further developed the ability to comprehend the meaning of a series of actions. Thus, a child of this age is better able to understand a thorough preparation for surgery or procedures, including all of the steps entailed in the process. A child of this stage is also for the first time capable of placing objects in an orderly sequence, arranging a set of sticks in order of increasing length, for example.

The increasing ability to think logically, as well as the new capacities for sequencing and imposing order are reflected in the play of these children. Games and other activities founded upon rules predominate. Secret clubs are established, based upon well planned charters. Teams are formed, and group activities become more competitive than in previous years.

Formal Operational Stage

The final of Piaget's four stages of intellectual growth is reached at approximately 12 years of age and characterizes adult thought. The direct actions which were necessary to develop the thought processes of children have been internalized. No longer must the individual rely upon the presence of physical objects to demonstrate logical thought. Those persons in the formal operational stage of development are now capable of abstract thought. A problem can be formulated, hypotheses generated, and various solutions explored, all in the mind of the individual without resorting to physical action. An adolescent may, for example, attempt to climb a steep rock ledge. Before doing so, the adolescent notes all possible routes, assesses benefits and dangers of each (visualizing places to stop and foreseeing rock slides or dead end paths), determines equipment needed, if any, and finally selects an opportune time to begin the adventure. The early play experiences of this individual's past, in the course of which new information was assimilated and accommodations made in old patterns of thought, have helped transform the prelogical thought of those early years into the abstract thinking needed to plan this climb so carefully.

Increased intellectual capabilities allow adolescents to specialize in their recreational activities, becoming expert in fields such as electronics, music, art, mechanics, and others requiring a high degree of abstract thought. New intellectual powers are also used to enhance and perfect activities previously adopted. The infusion of new strategies improves athletic performance; the ability to anticipate outcomes is beneficial to most pursuits.

Strictly speaking, Piaget considers play to be pure assimilation. That is, the child alters reality to fit into pre-existing modes of thought, regardless of the properties of the situation or materials involved. Thus, a child may take a wooden block and transform it into a car, despite its lack of wheels, doors, or a driver. Such play is said to serve a compensatory function. For example, Piaget (1962) describes his daughter's play as she pretends to carry her newborn cousin after being warned not to touch the baby. Activity of this sort "enables the child to relive his past experiences and makes for the satisfaction of the ego rather than for its subordination to reality (p. 131)." In other words, play enables the child to distort possibly upsetting aspects of reality into more agreeable patterns. In this respect Piaget's view of play closely corresponds to that of Erikson (see "Play and Emotional Development" in this chapter). In the preceding discussion a somewhat broader definition of play was adopted, roughly corresponding to the child's active manipulation of and interaction with the physical and social environment.

Play and Social Development

Even as play provides a mechanism for promoting physical and intellectual growth and development, it also serves an important role in the child's development as a social being. Much of the play of a very young child is isolated, mainly concentrating on the child's own body and immediate surroundings. Early interaction with others is typically limited to adults, who engage the infant in play experiences of various types. When other children are first discovered, they may be explored as if they were another fascinating toy, with one young child feeling, poking, and handling the other. A moment later such children will ignore each other. Social interaction with peers is limited at this age, although this may be attributed more to lack of opportunity than to inability to respond to infant playmates. Recent studies have indicated playful interactions among infant peers prior to their first birthday (Mueller & Vandell, 1979).

With time and opportunity, however, children will begin to regularly play next to each other, although minimal verbal communication may take place. Eventually the play activity becomes the source of limited interaction, as children comment on each other's play. This limited interaction leads to cooperation among playmates, who increasingly organize their play into more complex forms.

A categorization of social participation, based on the play behavior of children, was first suggested by Parten (1932) and is still widely used in play research. Parten's six categories suggest a progression from solitary behavior, through limited interaction to more complex cooperative play. While recent research has challenged the categorization of solitary play as an immature activity (Moore, Evertson & Brophy, 1974; Rubin, Maioni & Hornung, 1976), the play behavior of children is still seen to advance from parallel activity, to associative and, finally, cooperative play. Parten's categories are as follows:

UNOCCUPIED BEHAVIOR. Children demonstrating this behavior seem not to be playing—watching, instead, whatever strikes them as interesting. In the absence of a focus of interest, they will manipulate their own bodies, remain stationary, or move to a different location.

ONLOOKER PLAY. Although not actively involved in play themselves, onlookers focus their attention on the play activity of others, remaining close to the participating group. Onlooker play differs from unoccupied behavior in that the onlooker is consciously observing specific play of others, rather than merely attending to the most exciting stimulus at a given time.

SOLITARY INDEPENDENT PLAY. Children engaging in this play do so alone, using materials different from other children in the vicinity. No effort is made by the independent player to interact with others. Although Parten (1932) believed solitary play to be an immature form of play, recent studies have indicated that children of all ages engage in this behavior and that much of this activity is intellectually quite advanced.

PARALLEL ACTIVITY. This play is characterized by children playing in the same area with like materials, but with each using the materials in an independent manner. No attempt is made to alter the play of others. As Parten (1932) states, the child "plays *beside* rather than *with* the other children (p. 262)."

ASSOCIATIVE PLAY. In associative play, children interact with each other while engaged in a common activity. Materials may be exchanged, and there may be some attempts to control or limit participation, but the play is not organized. The group shares no common goal. According to Parten (1932), children participating in such play "do not subordinate their individual interests to that of the group; instead each child acts as he wishes (p. 264)."

COOPERATIVE OR ORGANIZED SUPPLEMENTARY PLAY. In this form of play, a group goal has been developed. The children involved may be producing an artwork, playing a formal game, or dramatizing a situation, e.g. playing "doctor" or "house". Play is usually directed by one or two of the players and is characterized by differentiation of roles. Entry to the group is controlled by its members.

By the time children enter elementary school, their play activities typically involve at least some organized cooperative play with other children. Such play becomes increasingly complex and structured as children move into the concrete operational stage of development, characterized by a preoccupation with rule-making. Cooperative play is a vehicle through which the school-age child explores potential friendships and solidifies their bonds.

Interactive skills developed through cooperative play during the school-age years are of crucial importance as children move into adolescence. The nature of the cooperative play is altered in the adolescent years, with recreational activities supplanting dramatic play and various games; but the social implications of such interactions remain highly important. Participation in groups gives the adolescent a sense of belonging, a feeling of extreme import during this peer-conscious age. Recreational activities centering around a given theme or skill, e.g. athletics, photography, music, etc., help the adolescent define his or her interests and explore possible future occupational roles. Thus, group activities can assist the adolescent struggling with questions of self-identity. Cooperative interaction further allows the adolescent, who is attempting to deal with biological maturation, and opportunity to come into contact with potential partners and explore new behaviors in the role of a sexual being.

Throughout all of childhood, from the earliest contact with other humans to the threshold of adult life, play experiences enable people to come together and, in the course of a pleasurable activity, learn how to function with others. This is not a conscious goal of the play, but rather a by-product, emerging as the child discovers that the satisfaction derived from play is heightened as it is enjoyed and shared with others.

Play and Emotional Development

The idealized, carefree period of childhood exists mainly in the minds of adults who have forgotten the difficulty and pain associated with this time of life. Fears, fantasies, and insecurities continually accompany children as they proceed toward maturity. Inner conflicts arise as they confront changes in themselves and the surrounding world. As Erikson (1963) has said, "To grow means to be divided into different parts which move at different rates (p. 211)." The child's attempts to synthesize the various facets of growth and development, while maintaining a healthy emotional balance, is facilitated by the child's ability to resolve emotional conflicts through play.

Whether in a structured setting such as a psychologist's office or hospital playroom, or in the informal atmosphere of a child's own room at home, the therapeutic nature of play reveals itself. The child busily acts out scenes, manipulates play materials, and draws pictures with accompanying stories. These and other activities allow a child to confront and struggle with problems in a safe environment, enabling the child to better deal with the problems in the more threatening "real world." Therapeutic play offers the child an opportunity for increased *self-expression*, thereby externalizing feelings previously hidden away, and for *mastery* of difficult situations.

Self-Expression

For younger children, feelings engendered by a threatening situation will far exceed the child's ability to express them. The limited vocabulary of a toddler cannot describe the difference between feelings such as fear, mild displeasure, and intense hatred. Yet such feelings can be communicated by the way a child plays, as revealed by a two-year-old boy and his teddy-bear companion observed in a hospital playroom: With a stern look the child placed the bear in a chair in an isolated corner of the playroom, in obvious disapproval of some prior wrong-doing by the bear. As a nurse entered the playroom to have the child return to his room for examination by his physician, the boy raced to retrieve his teddy. His reluctant stance and his vise-like clinging to the bear told the nurse of the child's fear. The sensitive nurse reflected the child's mood, commenting that he looked frightened. By doing so, the nurse labeled a feeling for the child, thereby increasing his awareness of it.

Upon returning to the playroom, the child's slamming to the floor of the bear and his vigorous, although only moderately successful, kicking of the same demonstrated his extreme anger over some aspect of the examination.

Often a child who may possess adequate verbal skills is reluctant to talk about thoughts or feelings that are excessively threatening or socially unacceptable. Through play, however, particularly in the presence of an accepting and encouraging adult, such feelings may be released. At times, only the emotion itself will be released, as in the case of Josh's destruction of the tower with the bean bag, described at the beginning of this chapter. Continued observation of the child's play, however, will generally yield clues as to possible sources of conflict in the child's life.

The frequency with which a theme enters a child's play corresponds to the intensity of the conflict in the child's life (Erikson, 1963, p. 217). For example, a child who is experiencing a major conflict over having been left at the hospital by parents may give evidence of this conflict in various play settings and with several play media. A family picture might be drawn in which the child omits himself or herself. A set of dolls may be manipulated in a manner that rejects one of them. The child may, in fact, "turn the tables" and reject or abandon other people in the hospital, ordering a nurse to leave the room or frightening another patient by saying that he or she has been abandoned. In isolation, each of these activities might be considered insignificant, but closer observation uncovers a recurrent theme indicative of the fear a child feels.

Several activities commonly encouraged at home, school, or in the hospital offer excellent opportunities for self-expressive play. Doll play and dramatic play allow the child to create scenes and characters to express ideas or situations which present difficulties for the child. Artwork permits the child to vent feelings through physical activity, as well as through the content of the finished product. In a similar manner, making music or moving to that created by others enables a child to release and express conflictual emotions.

Mastery

Many of the conflicts and bitter feelings which arise in the life of children can be traced to the helplessness and powerlessness they feel in this world dominated by those larger than they. Adults tell children where they may go and when, further dictating which of a myriad of attractive objects may be explored in each given setting. At times the passive position of a child is acutely painful. Traumatic changes occur over which the child has no control, but through which the child must, nevertheless, suffer. Parents may divorce, a new child may enter the family, or the child may have to go to the hospital.

In the security of a play setting the child is permitted to regain the power necessary to cope with conflicts of a large or seemingly trivial nature. In play the child rules, becoming the active initiator of events rather than their passive victim. Children who have been forced to eat certain foods or go to bed at what seems to them an unnaturally early hour may, in a play setting, issue similar orders to their smaller companion, stuffed animals or dolls.

The child who faces a frightening event may use the play setting as a laboratory to test and rehearse the impending experience. Preschoolers may construct a make-believe classroom and play going to school, in a sense practicing for and mastering the upcoming activity. Children fearful of separation from parents can gain a sense of mastery over their terror by playing peek-a-boo or "going bye-bye." Through such activities the child adopts the active role, initiating the separation in a comfortable setting, thereby achieving control in an otherwise powerless situation.

These uses of play in maintaining emotional equilibrium are of particular importance to children facing the rigors of hospitalization. But the child life worker must remain aware of the paramount importance of play in all areas of a child's development, in order to promote effectively the growth of the whole child. In the next section, the specific uses of play by the hospitalized child will be examined in greater detail.

THE HOSPITALIZED CHILD'S PLAY

In the course of a normal day of play, children will engage in a number of different play experiences, which provide exercise for all areas of development. One minute the play is vigorous, but soon the child is content to leaf through a book. Emerging from the literary solitude, the child seeks the company of others, but is temporarily rebuked in efforts to join a preexisting play group. The child returns to solitude, organizing a play group from cooperative stuffed animals. Fortified by the success of this venture, the child returns to the play group and this time is readily accepted.

The situation described above has a number of highly desirable characteristics which promote healthy play. The child has access to a variety of materials designed to exercise the child's mind and body. Others are available with whom the child may play if so desired. Movement among the activities is fluid and unfettered, except for the structure imposed by the players themselves.

The event of hospitalization seriously threatens the quality of play and the extent to which the child may engage in it. Since play is so important to the growth of the child, to impede play is to discourage normal development. As discussed earlier, the child's physical condition may inhibit active, strenuous play. The child who must remain in bed or who is encumbered with an IV, cast, or other restraint is less readily able to engage in physical activities. These same inhibitors further threaten the social development of the child. Children confined in isolation rooms or receiving fluids from two IV's obviously are less able to move among different groups of children than the nonhospitalized child described above. Sometimes children who are more mobile despite restraints are reluctant to play with others, fearing that their condition makes them "different" from their playmates.

While the hospital is a place of potentially great intellectual stimulation for children, unless encouraged to interact with the novel aspects of the environment (through direct manipulation of materials and by asking questions), they will not derive this benefit. In fact, hospitalization can have a negative effect on the child's intellectual growth.

Conflicts which are common in the normal growth of the child are even more prevalent among hospitalized children who must deal with pain, separation, and much that is unfamiliar. The need to express these feelings and attain mastery over them through play experiences, so necessary for all children, reaches critical importance in the life of the hospitalized child.

Guiding the Play of Hospitalized Children

With this knowledge in mind, several principles for providing play experiences for hospitalized children can be established to promote growth in all areas:

Physical Development

(1) The child life worker should provide play activities commensurate with the child's level of development and medical condition. For example, the fact that a toddler has an IV in his or her hand does not necessarily mean that this child should not be allowed to walk or play in the playroom. If medically permissable, the child should be allowed to explore the playroom, under the watchful eye of an attendant.

(2) Activities should be adapted to the physical abilities of the child.

Children can engage in a number of activities normally requiring mobility and dexterity, despite temporary or permanent limitations, if the activities are properly adapted. Children can engage in a game of catch from a bed or a wheelchair. If the child has difficulty holding the ball, a larger ball or one with a different texture may be substituted. Children who have difficulty manipulating their fingers to catch the ball might use a special Velcro mitt and ball set.

(3) The play setting and materials should be adapted to allow for participation by those with physical limitations. Areas for play should be accessible to those children who must remain in wheelchairs or beds. Sand and water tables, as well as areas for artwork, should be planned to allow participation by these children.

Social Development

(1) Adequate, accessible space should be provided to allow patients to gather for play and interaction. Pediatric units serving adolescents as well as younger children may need separate areas for differing age-groups.

(2) The child life staff and other personnel should encourage contact among patients. Whenever medically possible, children should have opportunities for interaction with peers, in the individual rooms of the children or in the playroom.

(3) Group activities should be structured by the child life department to facilitate group interaction. For younger children this might mean group games or art projects, while older patients would participate in activities such as discussion groups.

Intellectual Development

(1) Stimulating activities should be provided for all age-groups. These activities need not be limited to the playroom. "Busy box" activity centers can be installed on walls in the hallways or individual rooms. A hospital newspaper, complete with roving reporters, can be a stimulating and involving affair for children at many levels of intellectual development.

(2) Direct exploration of the unique aspects of the hospital environment should be encouraged. Explanations of equipment should be given on a level appropriate to the age of the children. All safe equipment should be handled by the children; questions should be welcomed. Tours to other interesting parts of the hospital, such as the laboratory, laundry room, switchboard, or kitchen can be arranged.

(3) The child life department should coordinate efforts with the school program and insure that every child's schooling continues appropriately.

Emotional Development

(1) Provide materials conducive to self-expression and allowing the child to achieve mastery. These materials would include dolls, puppets, dramatic props, art materials and musical instruments.

(2) Be open and nonjudgmental of the child's play. Children may express feelings which are terribly frightening to them, such as hating their parents or wishing to kill a nurse. The child life worker should communicate to children that their feelings are accepted and understood, and that such feelings are not unusual. If one tries to talk the child out of his or her feelings ("You don't really hate that nurse"), the child will perceive that such thoughts are unacceptable, suppress them, and feel abnormal for having conceived them.

(3) Reflect the child's feelings through summarization of thoughts expressed or by labelling feelings expressed nonverbally. When a child acts as Josh did (see opening section of this chapter), stomping heavily, kicking toys, and growling, it is appropriate for the child life worker to comment that the child seems angry about something. This places a name on the child's emotion and helps to focus consideration on the elements producing it.

(4) Ask questions which probe the feelings of the children. If a child is playing doctor and in the process gives a doll a shot, the child life worker may ask the young doctor, "How does your patient feel about having a shot?" The child's answer may well reveal much about the way he or she perceives injections.

It should be noted that the categorization of activities as physical, social, intellectual, or emotional is rather arbitrary, and has been adopted for the sake of analysis to delineate the various aspects of a child's growth with which the child life worker must be concerned. Certain activities which seem principally to exercise the physical child may, in fact, do more for a child's intellectual growth. Other activities, which seem purely diversional in nature, can become the catalyst for emotional growth. Ultimately it is the child who will choose how the activity will be pursued.

One child life worker, for example, found that a group of three boys was interested in making a puzzle which, when constructed, would reveal the picture of several super-heroes. This was presumably a purely diversional form of recreation which the child life worker pursued in order to strengthen his relationship with the boys. As the figures began to take shape on the table in front of them, the child life worker asked who the boys would choose to be, if they could become one of the comic book heroes. Jeff, whose head was still wrapped in a large dressing from his brain surgery, picked the character who could make himself invisible. Scott, who had suffered injuries in a 20-foot fall from the path he was walking with his Scout troop, chose a hero who could stretch his body to infinite lengths, extending his reach wherever he pleased. Timmy, who was confined to a wheelchair, selected a character who could fly. It was soon apparent that each child had chosen a hero with characteristics important to each because of his particular condition. Thus an opportunity developed from what seemed to be a strictly diversional pursuit, to discuss the concerns of the boys relating to their medical conditions.

Coping with Emotional Conflicts through Play

Since the emotional concerns of children are so acute during hospitalization and psychological health so vulnerable, it is important to understand better how the child uses play during this stressful period to cope with conflict. In preceding sections the role of play in the emotional growth of the child has been discussed. The form which this play takes in the hospital will now be examined in more detail.

Normalization of the Situation

Through hospitalization the child is extracted from an accustomed home setting and forced to deal with the unfamiliarity of strange new surroundings. Child life staff and other hospital personnel can do much to reduce the unfamiliarity by preparing the child for the event, encouraging parental participation, and making the hospital environment more home-like. While the staff is making such efforts, the child is busy at play, attempting to normalize the new setting. Familiar toys and games from home are helpful, but the child may prefer to find the materials available at the hospital.

As a means of settling in, children may arrange their toys on shelves, unpack suitcases, and load up on supplies from the playroom. Children often decorate their own rooms, frequently drawing pictures of family, friends, and home. Such artwork serves the dual purpose of claiming new territory in the hospital, while being a reminder of the child's place in the nonhospital world.

The discovery that they can play in the hospital is, in itself, reassuring to the children. It reduces the foreign flavor of the environment and allows the child to mobilize other play-related coping mechanisms. In fact, some well-planned children's hospitals were designed so that the first thing the child sees when he or she steps out of the elevator into the nursing unit is a bright, inviting playroom.

Mastery through Play

Much of what children are asked to do in the hospital requires them to be passive. They must hold still for examinations, procedures, and injections. Often they are restricted to bedrest or told to remain in their rooms. The millions of dollars of equipment they view is designed for use *on* them, not *by* them. Unless the child is extremely ill, the passive nature of this role will be difficult to accept. Frustrations generated by this condition can be alleviated through the child's play activities, as the passive recipient turns active.

Through the manipulation of dolls and puppets, the child may act out and gain mastery over the frightening prospect of separation. The child dragging a noisy pull toy ceaselessly around the hallways may, through this play, be dealing with such fears. The child controls the toy's string and is reassured by the noise that the toy is close at hand. Only when the child decides to let loose of the string will there be a separation.

Naturally, much of the anxiety experienced by hospitalized children arises from the frightening nature of medical equipment and treatments. The child with such anxiety will seek opportunities to gain mastery over this equipment, exploring it thoroughly and using it on others. Some children may find the actual equipment too threatening to handle, preferring miniature reproductions which are more easily manipulated and dominated. Real equipment, as well as smaller replicas, should be readily available for children's play.

Children may also wish to play through events which seem particularly frightening. One hospitalized boy was seen mentally rehearsing for an upcoming injection, each run-through climaxing with a scream as he pinched himself. Another girl practiced walking to the elevator on which she would go to surgery the following morning. Through such play the children were preparing themselves and obtaining a form of mastery over a scary event. At other times children may dramatize frightening events *after* they occur, almost always reversing roles with the doctors and nurses who inflicted the fearsome experiences on them. By role reversal such as this, children identify with the powerful figures in their experiences and attempt to undo the trauma of situations in which they perceive themselves as having been the victim.

Self-Expression through Play

The child who enters a hospital and experiences all that is scary and new will undoubtedly generate a whole new wave of feelings centered around these events. Through play the child has the opportunity to express these feelings. The way in which materials are handled, facial expression, and the content of dramatic play all function as vehicles for the communication of feelings. The presence of a child life worker or other staff member sensitive to these messages facilitates the reception of the communication and allows the staff to respond in a sensitive manner.

STAFF RESPONSE TO PLAY

From the moment a child arrives at the hospital, the need for play is present. Through play children seek to reconstruct their world, normalize their surroundings, gain a sense of dominance over the frightening, and express their often scary thoughts. Recognizing the ever-present nature of play, the child life worker and other members of the health care team can make use of it in performing their functions and in minimizing the danger of psychological damage to the children.

Monitoring Regression

Through observation of the child's play, the child life worker can monitor a child's regression to earlier levels of development. One seven-year-old who had been described by her mother in the admission interview as an eager group player was observed detaching herself from group situations. Much of her time was spent in parallel play activities or isolated, independent play. Although some regression is expected as a means of coping with the stress of hospitalization, it should not be encouraged. The child life worker in this case concentrated on structuring activities to support the girl's return to group participation.

Understanding Fears and Feelings

As mentioned previously, children will reveal feelings in their play, even when no one is present to observe the play. At times the feelings will be expressed in an inappropriate manner—threatening other children, damaging property, or endangering the child's own health. Realizing that children will continue to express their feelings, though perhaps hidden under a cloak of play, the child life worker must

    (1) see that such expression finds an appropriate vehicle (e.g. Josh's toppling the tower instead of terrorizing toddlers),

    (2) seek to understand the source of such feelings.

The process of understanding the source of feelings expressed through play is well illustrated by the case of Frank L.:

It was easy to see that 11-year-old Frank was upset. Unlike some children who fear expressing their secret wishes to kill or injure the medical staff, Frank was most willing to make his plans public. A hernia repair was scheduled for the following day, but the staff now discussed the possibility of cancelling it, for Frank stood on a chair in the corner of the room threatening various forms of violence to the unsuspecting lab tech who had arrived to take a blood sample. Realizing that it would take a small army to hold down the husky youth, the technician beat a quick retreat and suggested someone call the child life worker.

Linda, the Child Life Specialist, decided to introduce needle play to Frank to observe his response. Frank seized upon the opportunity, eagerly learning how to draw sterile water into a syringe. A willing doll was enlisted as a patient. Frank posed the needle over the doll's arm and, with a sneer, said, "And now I jab it down into the bone!"

Linda allowed Frank to repeat his violent jabbing of the doll, since he was being careful not to hurt himself. While watching Frank's actions, Linda recalled that Frank had spent some time earlier in the day waiting for an X-ray in a waiting area which also serviced the out-patient department. During that time a leukemia patient, whom Linda had known from previous hospitalizations, had been in one of the examining rooms for a bone marrow examination. The young girl generally found the "bone marrows" extremely terrifying and painful. Linda wondered if Frank perhaps associated this girl's procedure, which he could not have helped but overhear, with the needle work he would experience in the hospital.

When Linda asked Frank if anything had happened this morning when he went to get his X-ray, Frank related the story of the screams coming from behind the closed door. Frank had asked a receptionist why the girl was crying and was told that she was having a special "blood test" in which the doctors stuck a needle into the bone!

Once the source of Frank's anxiety over the blood test was revealed, Linda could begin to reassure Frank that his test was quite different and could prepare him for the event. This she did through play and by allowing Frank to observe a similar test performed on an older patient.

Enhancing Communication

Not all children are as willing to show their emotions or to express their feelings as Frank. Some children become quite shy, and are initially reluctant to trust the child life worker or others. Such children will still possess the urge to play. By introducing play activities and letting the child decide what he or she wants to do, the child life worker will be able to build a relationship and gain the child's trust. To pressure the child into a certain activity or to rush to impose a relationship before the child is ready may have the opposite effect, causing the child to withdraw further.

Through the sensitive use of play activities the child may begin to communicate with the child life worker. For the child who finds it difficult to talk directly about feelings or concerns, puppet or doll play may be introduced. While it may be difficult for a child to tell the child life worker how much he or she hates the hospital, a Cookie Monster® puppet or teddy bear may do so with impunity. In a similar manner, a child may refuse to answer the questions of a child life worker, but will do so when rephrased through the mouth of a Snoopy® doll.

Artwork may also be used as a means of enhancing communication. If a child has drawn a picture, the child life worker may ask the artist "tell me about your picture." Such phrasing allows the child to tell a story about the picture, while the hackneyed "What is it?" unnaturally forces the child to place a single label on the piece. Through talking about their pictures, children become aware of the subconscious conflicts which appear in their work.

Other art media can also encourage communication. One boy's long-hidden fears were revealed through the figures he formed from Play-Doh®: Five-year-old Barry had been too cooperative since his arrival in the hospital on Thanksgiving Day. He had fractured his leg in a fall from a chair and had been in traction for nearly three weeks. His uncomplaining adjustment to the immobilization caused staff to wonder if he weren't suppressing his anger and fears.

As Barry molded figures from the Play-Doh, the child life worker, whom Barry had grown to accept, asked Barry to tell him about the figures. Becoming increasingly agitated as he molded and kneaded the substance, Barry formed the figure of a boy. Taking a knife, he slashed the boy apart, saying, "The doctors did that to him!"

"Oh, why did they do that to him?"

"Because they're mean and they don't like him," was his reply. Smashing the fragments of the boy into a wad, Barry molded something that looked like a stocking. Again he destroyed it with the knife.

"That's Christmas! The doctor's took it away 'cause they don't like the boy!"

Although it was yet a week before Christmas and Barry would almost certainly be going home for the holidays, he was unconvinced. Barry's play had two important effects: (1) he had a chance to release the anger which the staff had long suspected, and (2) he made his concerns about Christmas known so that he could receive reassurance from the staff that his condition would not prevent the coming of Christmas.

Education and Preparation

An increasing number of enlightened pediatric facilities are recognizing the importance of preparing children for hospitalization and the various procedures they will encounter. The quality of preparation programs varies greatly, however, with too many relying solely on the verbal transmission of information to the patient. This runs contrary to our knowledge of how young children learn, for they gain their knowledge through active participation with concrete materials. Young children will not comprehend the significance of long lists enumerating the order of upcoming events. Explanations devoid of pictures or models will have little meaning for the children and may, in fact, be counterproductive by allowed the children to conjure up frightening images of the material discussed.

Children in the hospital set about trying to educate themselves through their play. A two-year-old girl picks up a needle-less syringe and with the eye of a practiced scientist assays its texture, weight, taste and mechanical properties, in the process convincing herself that it isn't really the monstrous animal it appeared to be. Another child watches with keen interest — and no little pleasure — as a blood pressure cuff inflates under his insistent pumping of the rubber bulb.

The child life worker and others involved in preparation must recognize the importance of play in a child's learning if effective preparation is to occur. Active, involved preparation of young children by the child life worker has several important benefits. First, it imparts information to the children in a meaningful form. Secondly, it allows the children to concentrate on areas of particular concern. A child, for example, may be terribly concerned about the catheter tubing used on the preparation doll. The child life worker who has allowed the child to be an active participant will easily detect the anxiety and deal with this specific concern. If the child were not involved in an active way, the discomfort with the catheter might never have been detected.

Finally, by allowing the child to play with the materials and act out the procedures, potential misconceptions can be more readily revealed. The child who administers a preoperative injection to a doll, saying that it is necessary because the doll was bad, demonstrates a misunderstanding of the purpose of injections. This important information might never have been discovered had the preparer merely offered verbal information, followed by the obligatory "Any questions?"

Summary

Play is an inextricable part of the child's life, enjoying predominance over all other waking activities. When children arrive at the hospital, their world may be shaken and their security threatened, but they nevertheless come prepared to play. The child life worker can ease a child's emotional adjustment to the hospital and minimize the hazards to normal growth and development by fostering an environment conducive to play, cultivating the child's natural urge to play, and providing a balanced program of activities.

CHAPTER 5

IMPLEMENTING A PLAY PROGRAM

PLAY THROUGHOUT THE HOSPITAL

One notices the difference almost immediately. It's not an unnerving difference, but a warm, reassuring one, nearly imperceptible, yet pervading the atmosphere: The expected silence is replaced by subtle layers of competing sounds. Hand-clapping music issues from the playroom. The bell of a tricycle patrols the hallway. Concerned voices engage in a debate of the rules of a board game.

The walls, the desk at the nurses' station, the shelves in the patient's rooms—all testify to the presence of active children. Papers covered with designs, sprawling patterns of color, and drawings of families and animals form a mosaic on the available wall space. From one of the pictures, a crudely-drawn face, its tongue sticking out, stares at passers-by. Below this head are scrawled the words, "ROGER SAYS THE HOSPITAL STINKS." Small clay figures, multicolored woven fabric, and a fantastic structure made of buttons, spools, rocks, and yarn are also in view.

In a room near the elevator a group of adolescents interrupts a pool game to listen intently as one of them talks. A burst of laughter erupts from the group as the speaker concludes his story.

The casual visitor to a hospital unit such as this is readily aware of the integration of play into hospital activities. All ages of children and adolescents are involved and busy. Some of the play experiences have a definite structure, such as the preschool music session in the playroom. Other activities, though more spontaneous and informal, are nevertheless promoted and encouraged by the careful planning of the child life staff. Adolescent gatherings and impromptu play sessions can occur because attractive materials are provided and adequate space is made available.

The opportunity for play experiences does not stop upon leaving the inpatient pediatric unit. A visit to other areas of the hospital with which children have contact reveals similar activity. A dozen children in the outpatient pediatric clinic pursue a variety of activities, alone or in small groups. A boy constructs a tower from oversize wooden blocks, straining on his toes to add just one more. Several parents watch with their children as the child life worker mixes a batch of finger paint. The parents are provided with written instructions so that they may repeat the process at home. A child life trainee plays doctor with a girl who awaits her own examination.

In the X-ray department, a four-year-old girl in Snoopy pajamas pushes a truck across the carpet to a child life volunteer, while her mother reads a pamphlet on X-ray procedures. Across the hall in the emergency room waiting area, a boy, whose sister fractured her arm in a fall from her bike, furiously scribbles on a sheet of paper.

The critical role of play in the child's growth and development, and especially in the child's emotional adjustment to the hospital experience, was discussed in the previous chapter. To benefit hospitalized children, this knowledge must be transformed into action through the establishment of a well-planned play program.

SCOPE OF THE PLAY PROGRAM

As in the setting just described, the child life play program should provide activities for all age-groups. From infancy through adolescence, each age-group has characteristic problems in facing illness and hospitalization. These commonly-held problems are modified and compounded by other concerns unique to each child. Furthermore, every child struggles with the normal developmental tasks of his or her age. Play and recreational opportunities provide all ages with a vehicle for dealing with emotional stress and for continuing the encounter with developmental concerns, despite the disruption of hospitalization. Even as the preschooler profits from doctor play, so the adolescent gains from discussion groups and informal activities in the teen lounge.

The play program should reach all areas of the hospital where children are required to spend time. The anxieties engendered by hospital experiences are not confined to the pediatric unit. Neither should the child's access to play be artificially demarcated in this manner. In fact, many moments of greatest stress for the child occur outside the pediatric inpatient unit. Too often during these stressful times, such as admission, X-rays, examinations, laboratory tests, and prior to induction of anesthesia, children are denied an opportunity to play because of lack of materials, space, and professional guidance. And thus they are denied one of the most therapuetic of activities at the very times they are in greatest need of it.

Other areas of the hospital serve children who are not admitted as inpatients, but who are nevertheless susceptible to the fears and anxieties inherent in any medical setting. Children may briefly visit the laboratory or X-ray department for medical procedures. Though not hospitalized, these children are still in need of (1) explanations concerning the environment and procedures, and (2) play experiences that will help them cope with their feelings.

The outpatient pediatric clinic, which is often the sole source of medical care for children, many of whom will later be hospitalized, should provide extensive play experiences for its visitors. Azarnoff and Flegal (1975) have discussed the importance of an outpatient play program:

> Although hospitalization adds the additional anxiety of separation from the family, the clinic may be frightening, too. The clinic remains a place in which children can perceive examinations and treatment procedures as invasive, threatening, and restrictive. Therefore, they need reassurance, information and autonomy in clinics as well as in hospitals, and both places need trained behavioral specialists to assist in pediatric work (p. 10).

By providing children with pleasurable and psychologically beneficial experiences through an outpatient play program, the child life department is helping them formulate positive attitudes toward medical care. Should these children later be hospitalized, the positive feelings nurtured in the clinic play program will facilitate their adjustment to the hospital environment.

Children who visit the emergency room of a hospital generally do so under the most trying of circumstances. With the sudden event of an illness or accident, the child is whisked off to this unusual place by anxious parents and is confronted by all of its strangeness without benefit of preparation for the experience. The opportunity to play while waiting, if the child is well enough, or to receive reassurance from a child life worker is important.

Brothers and sisters can also receive benefit from the child life play program in the emergency room. Frequently they accompany the ill or injured child, since the immediacy of the situation prevents parents from arranging for someone to stay with them. The sights and sounds of an emergency room can be quite intense for any observer, but especially so for young visitors who may already have begun to fantasize about the fate of a sibling taken out of their sight. Here, again, the child life play program can be of vital importance as frightened young children attempt to deal with their feelings.

Provision should also be made for the siblings of hospitalized children. These children may be integrated into the inpatient play program or play in the outpatient playroom. Ideally, a separate sibling play area can be established by the child life program to meet the unique needs of these children.

A comprehensive hospital play and recreation program, attending to the emotional and developmental needs of all children and adolescents throughout all areas of the facility, should be an ultimate goal of the child life department. To provide a narrower range of services denies support to children during what are frequently periods of high emotional risk, thereby leaving the children more vulnerable to psychological upset. Unfortunately, few institutions can readily implement such a comprehensive program, concentrating instead on the development of a few aspects of it.

Apportioning Limited Staff and Resources

Until sufficient staff and adequate play areas are available to meet the need for play throughout the hospital, some compromises and choices must be made in the allocation of child life services. The selection of areas and particular children to be served by the limited staff, a difficult and frustrating task, should be based on carefully formulated priorities derived from the perceived needs of the patients. The inpatient pediatric unit and the outpatient clinic are generally the first areas in which child life services are organized. As additional staff become available, services may expand to the emergency room and other waiting areas.

Prior to the full expansion of child life services to areas other than the pediatric unit and outpatient department, limited service may be arranged. For example, if many children are routinely admitted to the hospital at the same time of day, an inpatient child life worker might spend a few hours daily in that waiting area, helping children in their initial orientation. When services in other waiting areas are nonexistent, individual children may still receive attention. A child life worker, trainee, or volunteer might accompany children (particularly those for whom the experience may be difficult) to other areas of the hospital, such as X-ray. In smaller facilities, such as community general hospitals, whose individual departments serve limited numbers of children, the accompanying of individual children to these areas may be the only practical way of extending child life services to them.

The choice of which children should receive child life attention frequently remains, even after a limited number of areas for concentration have been established. The initial staffing of a child life inpatient program, for example, may be such that to serve all children adequately would be impossible. The child life staff must face the decision of extending some service to all children or more significant services to fewer children. This difficult professional decision should be made in consultation with other members of the health care team, and in consideration of other hospital services available to children and their families. If, for instance, Social Services provides an active program of support and consultation to families and Nursing provides an effective program of preoperative preparation, the child life staff may feel comfortable in concentrating on the preadmission tour and the play program, serving only as a resource person in other areas.

Priorities for Child Life Services

Unfortunately, in many hospitals an even more frustrating dilemma must be faced—what can be done if the hospital budget will not permit the hiring of adequate staff to service all inpatient units reasonably well? Does a limited, overworked staff try to provide a minimal level of service to all inpatients (thin coverage) or do they try to provide high quality child life services for certain patients or on a few nursing units and ignore the rest? As Carolyn Larsen (1980) points out, there is no easy way out of this dilemma. Some child life workers have taken the latter course—not attempting to serve all patients until adequate staff can be hired—reasoning that the hospital administration will more quickly feel the pressure to increase the department's budget if some units are not receiving any services. Other child life workers consider the withholding of services to be morally indefensible, arguing that the staff must do their best to serve all children, no matter how superficially. Most departments adopt a position that lies somewhere in the middle of these two extremes.

When attempting to identify those children most in need of child life services, the following factors should be considered:

Age of the Patient

Although children of all ages experience difficulty in adjusting to hospitalization, those from about seven months to three or four years of age are particularly vulnerable to psychological trauma. The services of the child life department, especially the play program, are highly important for children of this age.

High Risk Children

Other children outside the most vulnerable age-group may also be particularly susceptible to emotional distress, because of family situations or past experiences. Children who have had difficulty with a previous hospitalization or who have recently experienced a death in the family are among this group. Other factors such as parental marital problems, the birth of a sibling, or the inability of parents to visit call for increased vigilance by the child life staff.

Medical Condition

The condition for which children are admitted to the hospital, or the type of medical treatment they will receive, may indicate a special need for play and other child life interventions. Severe illnesses and extended hospitalization can heighten a child's anxiety and anger, thereby increasing the necessity for play experiences to assist the child in coping with these feelings. Children on bedrest, immobilized, or in isolation, and therefore unable to participate in normal group functions, should also receive special play attention to help them deal with the frustration aggravated by their condition.

It is not uncommon for a hospitalized child to be diagnosed as having a disease which will entail long-term changes in his or her life. The child with diabetes, for example, must face sometimes difficult alternations in diet and daily injections. A cancer patient may encounter the tribulations of severe chemical therapy, surgery, or amputation, and the ever-present prospect of death. The child life staff should use play to help children adjust to these radical changes and to build a trusting relationship which can offer great support to them.

Manifested Problems

It is inevitable that some children will experience severe difficulty adjusting to hospitalization even though their age, condition, or previous experiences have not suggested potential problems. Those children manifesting behavior which indicates the presence of problems should be considered high priorities for the attention of the child life staff.

At best, the process of setting priorities for which patients will receive concentrated child life interventions is flawed. Children who fall outside the categories listed above (for example, a school-age child briefly hospitalized for minor surgery) might receive only a small amount of professionally observed play. Such a child may, indeed, have experienced problems related to the hospitalization, problems which might have been resolved if the child had a greater opportunity to learn, gain mastery, and express feelings through play. If the difficulties did not surface until after the child had returned home, which is often the case, the necessity for increased child life intervention would have gone unrecognized. To minimize the possibility of missing such individuals, sufficient child life staff should be available to reach all children served by the hospital.

PROGRAM REQUIREMENTS

Staffing the Child Life Program

The question of staffing is a crucial one for child life programming. Operating an effective play program and attending to other emotional needs of children and their families require many hours of diligent work by properly trained professionals each day. The Association for the Care of Children's Health (ACCH) has published *Guidelines for the Development of Child Life Programs* (1980). Concerning the hours of program coverage, the guidelines state that, "A five day per week, eight hour per day program is considered minimal coverage. The evening hours and weekends have special strains that additional programming can help to relieve (p. 10)." An even stronger statement on extended coverage is contained in guidelines published by the Committee on Hospital Care of the American Academy of Pediatrics (1971): "The recreational program should operate on evenings and weekends, in addition to normal working hours. When possible, it should be extended to waiting and outpatient areas (p. 53)."

The truth of these statements is verified by a brief review of activities on a pediatric unit. Morning finds many anxious, ambulatory children awaiting surgery, with other patients also ready for play. Throughout the day children may experience long periods alone while parents are at work or are tending to siblings. During the afternoon and through the evening patients scheduled for surgery the following day arrive, needing play, reassurance, and preparation for forthcoming events. Although fewer children may be hospitalized on weekends, those who remain are generally hospitalized for longer periods or more severe conditions, and therefore are in special need of child life services. Since the emotional needs of children do not conform to a 40-hour work week, child life activity should not be limited to weekday hours.

The number of people required to operate an effective play program will vary with each setting, and is dependent on the breadth and depth of services offered by child life personnel. Several authorities have recommended a 1 to 15 ratio of child life staff to pediatric patients (Crocker, 1974; Azarnoff and Flegal, 1975). The American Academy of Pediatrics (1978) sets the following minimum standards:

> It is necessary for each pediatric unit, no matter how small, to have at least one employee whose sole function is recreation. Larger units should maintain a ratio of at least one paid employee for each 30 patients. This will still provide only minimal coverage and should be supplemented by volunteers (p. 53).

In its Position Paper (1979), the Child Life Activity Study Section of the Association for the Care of Children's Health set a 1:10 ratio of child life staff to pediatric patients. This figure, however, was not meant to imply that one child life worker per 10 patients would be working in the hospital at a given time but instead suggests that the entire child life staff (including coverage for evenings and weekends), when divided into the number of pediatric beds, would result in the 1:10 ratio.

Few hospitals presently can claim to meet these staffing standards. In a survey of members of the National Association of Children's Hospitals and Related Institutions, McCue et al. (1978) discovered that:

13% of the hospitals surveyed had fewer than 15 patients per child life staff member

47% of the hospitals surveyed had 15-40 patients per staff member

27% of the hospitals surveyed had 40-100 patients per staff member

13% of the hospitals surveyed had more than 100 patients per staff member.

It would appear that a ratio of 1:15 is a goal to work for, but that an absolute minimum of 1:20 or 1:25 might be a necessary compromise in many situations. Departments whose budgets will not allow more than one child life worker for 40-50 patients may need to consider restricting their services to fewer units until adequate staff can be hired.

Qualifications needed by child life staff have been outlined in detail in the Position Paper (1979) and *Guidelines* (1980) published by the ACCH. The reader is urged to consult both these documents for further information. In light of increased concern for establishing minimum standards for the preparation of child life personnel (Stanford, 1980), it can be anticipated that even more rigorous guidelines will be forthcoming.

Little can be said about basic salary figures for child life workers. The survey by McCue et al. (1978), conducted in the spring of 1976, revealed that salaries for program *directors* ranged from $4,944 per year to $24,000 per year. The researchers discovered that programs with larger staff seemed to have a somewhat higher rate of salary for the director, but that there did not seem to be any relationship between salary and either education or experience.

More recent data are presented by Mather and Glasrud (1980), who discovered that the average annual salary for 79 percent of the total program *staff* (as opposed to just the directors surveyed by McCue et al.) ranged from $10,000 to $14,000. Some hospitals attempt to keep salaries for beginning child life workers on a par with the salary figure for beginning school teachers in the local system. Other hospitals start child life workers at the same salary as they do registered nurses and occupational therapists. Generally, though, salaries fluctuate greatly from hospital to hospital, the most significant contributing factor being the state of the budget of the respective hospital.

Budget for the Child Life Program

Many of the child life programs presently in existence were established through grant money or with funds provided by an auxiliary or volunteer group. This funding has proven invaluable in introducing child life services to hospitals, which would then, when hospital personnel had seen the value of the services for themselves, begin to support the program through the regular hospital budget. The support of outside groups, according to Rutkowski (1978), accounted for an average of 21 percent of the budgets of the 120 child life programs he surveyed.

Whether or not a child life program should continue to rely on outside sources of funding is debatable. The child life Position Paper (ACCH, 1979) insists that the child life program be funded totally by the general hospital budget, the reasoning being that failure of the hospital to provide financial security leaves the child life program vulnerable to the caprices of the funding sources. It has been the experience of others in the field that even when a program is included in the general hospital budget, it is not invulnerable to the budget slashing that seems to be the inevitable result of inflation and other factors. In fact, to some in the field, it appears that a child life program may have a greater chance of financial survival if most of its funding comes from outside the hospital in the form of grants, donations, and fund-raising events.

The exact amount needed to operate a high quality child life program cannot be established with any certainty. Rutkowski (1978) found that of the programs that responded to his question about the amount of their budget, the average amount spent per bed per year was $754.52, and of that an average of 83 percent was devoted to salaries.

The ACCH *Guidelines for the Development of Child Life Programs* (1980) lists a number of categories which should be covered in the funding of the child life program. Among these are the following:

Salary and Benefits for Staff

Provisions should be made for sufficient staff, based on the size of the population served and the needs of the individual hospital. Salary and benefits should be comparable to those of other hospital employees with similar educational backgrounds and experience, i.e. social workers, school program teachers, etc.

Office Space, Equipment, and Supplies

An area for the child life staff to plan, confer, and prepare materials is essential. The child life budget should allow for basic office materials, copying expenses, and phone service. The staff should have access to secretarial service as needed.

Storage Facilities

An active group of children will demand massive amounts of play materials, some of which must be stored away when not in use, while others should be attractively displayed and readily available. In either case, shelves and lockable cabinets must be purchased along with other initial major investments for the play program.

Play and Recreational Equipment

A major investment must initially be made to furnish recreational and play areas. In addition to the major furnishings, a large stock of toys, games and consumable materials must be obtained. The annual budget of the child life department should allow for the purchase of additional major items as needed and should be sufficient to replace or repair older items. Funds should further provide for the replenishment of consumable items such as paper, paints, and other art materials.

Special Entertainment, Parties, and Events

Birthdays, holidays, and other important times all too often coincide with the hospitalization of the child. The child life staff must be aware of such special occasions and celebrate them accordingly, by decorating the playroom or the area around the celebrant's bed and organizing group parties. The budget should provide funds for these special events.

Travel and Conference Expenses

Conferences sponsored by the Association for the Care of Children's Health or other organizations interested in the well-being of children are excellent sources of new ideas and techniques. Through these meetings child life workers are able to meet with other professionals to discuss common problems and share successes. The child life budget should include funds sufficient to allow staff members to participate in such conferences.

Educational and Resource Materials for Staff

The budget should allow for the purchase of journals, books, and other new materials pertinent to the field of child life.

Teaching Materials for Students

Child life programs which serve as fieldwork centers for child life trainees or other students must have provision in their budget for reprinted articles, audiovisual materials and other items for the students' use.

As indicated by these categories, a major initial investment must be made for materials and equipment when instituting a child life program. An adequate ongoing budget is also necessary to support the program's activities.

Space Requirements

The amount and nature of the space allocated for children's play significantly influences the nature of the play program. A large, attractive activity area, subdivided into well-defined interest areas, encourages children to enter and participate, whereas a smaller or less accessible area discourages them. The importance of play in the child's adjustment to the hospital mandates the provision of ample space for play activities in locations convenient to the child. Each pediatric unit must have its own play area, large enough to accommodate group activities, while allowing space for other pursuits such as artwork, games, or reading. According to the Academy of Pediatrics (1978), an appropriate size for a playroom is 25 square feet per patient served.

Accommodating the Population Served

The types of activities available in each playroom should reflect the needs of the population served. Among the more common groups of pediatric patients are the following:

HETEROGENEOUS GROUPING. Many hospitals place children on a given pediatric unit without regard for their age or medical condition. The playroom on a unit such as this must provide activities to serve a broad range of children from infants to early adolescents.

GROUPING BY MEDICAL CONDITION. Larger facilities will frequently assign children to a given unit according to their medical condition or reason for admission, e.g. surgical, orthopedic, or neurological units. Ages will vary widely in such units, once again demanding an extensive selection of materials for children of differing age-groups. In addition to providing these materials, the child life staff should make accommodations based on the condition of the children. A more elaborate collection of preparation materials may be placed in a surgical unit playroom, for example, or special equipment may be installed to enhance patient mobility in the orthopedic unit playroom.

GROUPING BY AGE. Significant alteration in playroom design is possible when children are assigned to a pediatric unit according to their age. While a playroom designed for infants and toddlers would provide ample "child-proof" floor space for activities, an area for school-age children would allow for group activities and art projects.

In addition to a play area in each unit, space should be provided for the following facilities:

An Outdoor Play Area

Children normally have ready access to the world outdoors, playing in the warmth of the sun, catching snowflakes on their tongues, examining fallen leaves, or conducting insect safaris. Too often hospitalized children are denied these experiences, a condition which emphasizes the abnormality of their situation. In an outdoor play area (constructed on a fenced-in portion of the roof or at ground level) children may picnic, engage in group activities, tend gardens, or merely sit and appreciate the welcome change of scenery. An area such as this helps to lessen the schism between a child's life in the hospital and that in the outside world.

A Large Motor Area

The mere fact that a child is in the hospital does not necessarily mean that he or she is incapable of physical activity. Presurgical patients frequently crave the opportunity to run, pass a football, tumble on mats, or otherwise vigorously exert themselves. By doing so they can reassure themselves of the essential soundness of their bodies and can discharge anxieties generated by the impending events. Certain nonsurgical patients may also engage in vigorous activity while hospitalized. Diabetics who are having their insulin levels adjusted often experience large amounts of inactive time. Physical exertion not only provides these children with a pleasurable, familiar activity, it also allows physicians to obtain a more accurate picture of the activity level of the child outside the hospital. Thus, physicians can more precisely determine the insulin needs of the children.

An area for large motor activity need not be a gymnasium, but any area large enough (and safe enough) to accommodate a moderate run and the tossing of a ball. An outdoor area would accomplish this purpose during periods of cooperative weather. A large meeting area can be converted to this use when not otherwise occupied.

A Teen Lounge

Although a multi-age playroom can be constructed to accommodate infants through school-age children, its function should not be extended to serve adolescents. The stigma of playing with younger children (except when clearly part of an older brother or sister role) is far too threatening and demeaning for adolescents, and will surely result in their making only limited use of the area. A separate teen lounge should be established. If an adolescent unit exists, this is the proper place for the lounge. If, however, adolescents are hospitalized among several units, a central location for the lounge can be chosen, with patients being encouraged to make use of the facility. While a trip out of the unit to find recreation space may inhibit the play of younger children, adolescents welcome the opportunity for movement and appreciate the freedom and trust such an arrangement implies.

In recent years a number of older facilities, designed before the importance of play for hospitalized children was widely understood, have established child life programs. Adequate space for play activities is frequently a major problem. In some cases, the number of certified beds on a pediatric unit has been reduced, thereby freeing a room for play. Azarnoff and Flegal (1975) suggest that if no other room exists, a portion of a waiting area, the end of a hallway, or a portion of a large patient room can be used as a play space. Failing to obtain even this limited space, they propose greater reliance on a mobile play cart equipped with a variety of activities, and the use of individual patient rooms as centers of play. Despite the most severe physical space limitations, it is essential that children have ready access to play experiences.

PLAYROOM DESIGN

The precise design of any given playroom is dependent on a number of factors such as the amount of space available, the needs of the population serviced, and the personal taste and desires of the child life staff. When designing any hospital play area, several guidelines should be followed.

General Guidelines

(1) The design should provide for play opportunities when the area is unsupervised. This is particularly important for settings with limited child life staff. Children must have access to play materials on weekends, in the evenings, and at other times when a child life worker is not on duty in the playroom. Materials which present a particular danger to young children (because they are easily swallowed, exessively sharp, or otherwise potentially harmful) or materials which could be easily destroyed by young hands should be locked in cabinets when the playroom is unattended. Harmless materials appropriate for young children e.g. balls, blocks, dolls, small trucks, etc., should be kept available. Materials more appropriate to older children may be placed on open shelves out of the reach of younger explorers.

The use of a room divider provides another solution to the accessibility problem. Games with small parts, record players, paints, and other art materials may be kept in an area of the playroom which can be secured by means of a movable screen or other divider during nonsupervised hours, leaving the remainder of the room safe for children's play.

(2) General safety factors must be assessed. Electrical outlets should be positioned out of the reach of small children. Radiators must be covered. Sharp edges on furniture, door and cabinet handles, and railings must be eliminated. The path of opening doors should be examined to assess the risk of hitting an unaware child playing below eye-level.

(3) The playroom must be accessible by wheelchair or gurney. If necessary, ramps must be installed and doorways widened. Furniture within the playroom (water and sand tables, art tables, easels, etc.) should also be of a type which can accommodate less mobile patients.

(4) A variety of materials and areas should be available to provide children with a clear choice of activities. Whether a child prefers active involvement or a quiet, contemplative time, interaction with others or solitary exploration, the environment should reflect acceptance of this choice. A few boxes positioned in the corner can create a quiet nook

where children may leaf through books or assemble puzzles. A wooden stove and refrigerator in another corner invites children to join in dramatic play, while a large, unobstructed area elicits movement and physical activity.

The child life program goals of encouraging a child's normal development and facilitating emotional adjustment can be enhanced through careful attention to playroom design. The materials and equipment necessary for play change as a child grows and develops, and play areas for different age-groups should reflect this change.

Age-Specific Guidelines

Depending on physical space allowances and pediatric unit composition, a hospital may provide separate play space for each age-group or integrate the play of several ages in a single room. In either case, an understanding of the types of materials most beneficial to each is important in developing an intelligent design. The following suggestions may form the core of a single playroom design, or they can be combined to meet the needs of a heterogeneous patient population:

Designing Play Space for Infants

The young observer lies in her crib, fascinated by the marvels of this newly discovered world. Miniature bears suspended from strings dangle above her head, moving slowly in a circle to the sound of delicate musical notes. She extends an arm toward the objects, but retracts it when suddenly startled by a noise from the doorway. A smiling figure enters the room, addressing the infant in a quiet, yet animated fashion. Her brief cry of apprehension is stilled as she feels warm hands support her and nestle her softly on a shoulder.

Infants experience the world through their senses, watching, listening, and feeling, eventually developing a mental framework for understanding and predicting the outcome of events. To assure the continuation of this process while a child is hospitalized, the child life department must provide a stimulating environment for the child.

While many forms of stimulation can be provided to infants in their cribs (through interesting designs on the walls, mobiles, music boxes, toys of differing shapes and textures, etc.), these alone are inadequate. Infants need exposure to other humans, to be held, talked to and played with. They also need opportunities for physical exercise, developing the capacity for crawling, lifting themselves, and standing—necessary precursors to walking.

A play area for infants can offer the child these opportunities. Here a child life worker can introduce a variety of physical and sensory experiences to the child and involve parents in play activities which can be continued at home. Those infants too young or otherwise physically incapable of active involvement should be afforded the opportunity to observe playroom activity from an infant seat.

Lindheim, Glaser, and Coffin (1972) suggest the construction of a large play-pen type area with a soft, warm floor, free of all hazards, on which the infants may crawl. Several sturdy objects should be placed in this area for the infants to crawl around or to use for steadying as they lift themselves to wobbly legs. A few simple toys may be introduced to the area to enhance the exploration.

The boundaries of the crawling area can be defined by a low plexiglas wall. This construction allows the infants to peer at observers outside the area, and can offer further assistance in the child's early attempts to stand. A padded, sunken area in the floor, 12 to 18 inches below floor level, is an alternative, more sophisticated design for the crawling space.

If an entire area cannot be devoted to this purpose, several options exist. A portion of a large playroom can be "walled off" for this purpose, or, if space does not allow for a permanent area, large foam blocks can be positioned to form a temporary infant area in any location of sufficient size.

Designing Play Space for Toddlers and Preschoolers

The skills of children in this age group are rapidly advancing. Problems of mobility and navigation, which so recently seemed insurmountable, have been conquered. Few areas lie out of the reach of the increasingly agile child. Language develops from the babbling imitation of sounds, through recognizable words, to complete sentences. The child's play moves from isolation, eventually intermeshing with that of others. Although children of this age are moving toward autonomy in personal care and toilet training, they are still highly dependent on parents. Their emotions tend to be mercurial.

Designing play spaces for these children is a challenge. Much of the activity of this group, particularly among its younger members, will occur on the floor. As in the infant area, the floor should be warm, soft, and free of danger. From the base camp of the floor, numerous expeditions will be launched into the higher reaches of the play facilities. This urge to perfect new physical skills should be channelled in acceptable ways. Small slides and other low climbing devices should be available, with soft material, such as pillows or plastic-covered foam rubber underneath. Bookshelves and other high areas in the playroom should be examined for their accessibility to climbing. If such furnishings are, in fact, climbable and present an unreasonable risk to the climber, they should be removed or the design modified.

The urge to explore cabinets and storage spaces within reach is overwhelming to the toddler and preschooler. Rather than discouraging this curiosity in designing the play space, one should take advantage of it. Play materials which are unsafe or inappropriate for young children should not be stored in the playroom or, if no other storage space exists, must be carefully locked away. A host of other materials can be stored in low shelves readily available to the toddler or preschooler. By presenting the materials in this manner, the child life staff allows the child to make choices about activities, thereby encouraging the movement toward autonomy.

Messy play is a favorite of toddlers and preschoolers, and provisions should be made for it. An area of the playroom floor should be tiled for easy clean-up, and a sink should be available. Water tables, art tables, and easels of appropriate size should be a part of the playroom equipment.

As children begin playing together, and as their language becomes more refined, dramatic play emerges. A few props such as old clothing, play kitchen furniture and toy dishes enhance the play. Concerns arising from the hospital experience can find expression in a medical play corner of the playroom. Children provided with surgical caps, gowns, stethoscopes, and needle-less syringes need little encouragement to adopt the roles of doctor and nurse, commencing their practice on any willing doll or teddy-bear.

A final necessity for the toddler and preschooler play area is rapid access to toilet facilities. Controlling bodily functions takes practice before mastery is achieved. When heavily involved in play, children often ignore their bodies' signals, until a crucial moment. A toilet close at hand can save the child undue embarrassment and can minimize the interruption of play.

Designing Play Space for School-Age Children

The difference between the play of preschoolers and that of children of school age is largely one of quality rather than kind. Many of the activities engaged in by preschoolers, e.g., physical exploration, dramatic play, art work, etc., are continued during the school years, although the form and emphasis vary. The school-age child is a more social being who tends to organize groups to participate in play. Children of this age are interested in the perfection of skills acquired in earlier years. Whereas the preschooler engages in artwork for the sake of the process (feeling fingerpaint ooze between fingers, watching different colors trickle together on paper, or pounding clay, just because it feels good), the school-age child develops an interest in the product. More effort and time are devoted to each project or activity than in previous years.

Play spaces for grade school children should accommodate the changing emphasis of their play. The facility should include a large open area for group play, as well as an expanded art center. Lindheim et al. (1972) propose the construction of a multipurpose area which would allow for much group activity, including dining, as well as the leisurely completion of projects. Subdivision of the room, through screens or movable barriers, allows several different activities to occur simultaneously. If enough space and tables are available, projects in progress may be left out until completed. Lindheim et al. further suggest ample storage space for a variety of materials from which the children may serve themselves.

The greater sophistication of the play of school-age children calls for the introduction of more realistic props for dramatic play. In the medical play corner a wealth of new materials may be provided to enrich their play and greatly enhance their understanding of medical equipment. Instruments such as reflex hammers, otoscopes, blood-pressure cuffs and IV set-ups should supplement the stethoscopes, bandages, and other basic equipment. The children may also wish to play with doll-sized wooden hospital furniture available from commercial manufacturers.

Designing Recreation Facilities for Adolescents

Although infant, toddler and preschooler, and school-age play areas may, if necessary, be combined in one large room, the recreation space for adolescents should be separate. The needs of adolescents are considerably different from those of younger children. Hofmann, Becker and Gabriel (1976) note:

> the concerns and interests of teenagers in television viewing and record and radio listening are notoriously at variance with those of adults or children, as are their differences in other preferred leisure activities. To share recreational activities with older or younger patients may result either in the imposition of adolescent boisterousness upon those who may find this distressing or, alternatively, in depriving adolescents of activities they enjoy (pp. 93–94).

The adolescent lounge should be of moderate size, large enough to accept a pool or ping pong table, while allowing seating for a small group. As Hofmann et al. indicate, a TV and stereo should be available, with patients encouraged to bring in their records from home. The lounge should be located in an area where the noise will present little problem to other patients. Accoustical materials should be used in the design of the room to confine the sound as much as possible.

Lindheim et al. suggest the inclusion of a snack bar: "A modest hot plate and soft drink arrangement is enough, for more elaborate facilities would involve clean-up problems (p. 93)." They further propose that the furniture and decor of the lounge be changeable to allow each group of teenagers to rearrange the room to its own taste.

Hospitalized adolescents find themselves in a difficult position — beyond childhood, yet suspicious of the adult world. By providing a lounge area for their use, free of the stigma associated with the pediatric unit, the hospital demonstrates a sensitivity to their conflicts.

Inpatient Play in Other Areas

As critical as well-designed playrooms are to the success of the child life program, not all play activities occur there. The child life staff encourages play in individual rooms as a means of strengthening friendships among roommates and to insure that those who are less mobile have adequate access to play experiences.

At times the child life worker may structure individual play sessions with children in their own rooms, as in the case of children in isolation who can neither come to the playroom, nor participate in play through the visits of other patients. During these play sessions the child life worker should provide the child with ample opportunity to express frustrations engendered in the isolation experience and should offer reassurance to the child that the isolation is temporary. Many children may believe the condition to be a form of punishment. The child life worker should be alert for this possible misconception.

In addition to the play sessions, the child life worker can minimize the feelings of ostracism which an isolated child often feels by providing activities which can be done when alone, and by serving as a communication link between the child in isolation and other patients. Messages can flow in and out of isolation (verbally, if paper cannot be carried out) via the child life worker. If there is a telephone in the isolation room, the child life worker can arrange for other children to call in their greetings.

Activities of the inpatient child life program need not be confined to the nursing unit. Every hospital is filled with dozens of interesting places, among them the laboratory, laundry, and food preparation areas. Through field trips to departments such as these children gain a better understanding of the total operation of the hospital, making the whole experience more comprehensible. The need for blood samples, for instance, is more easily explained when a child is given the opportunity to see how specimens are analyzed or is allowed to look through a microscope. The arrival of a child's food tray takes on a new meaning after he or she has seen the kitchen in which it was prepared.

In a further effort to reduce the distinction between the hospital and nonhospital worlds, the child life program may sponsor activities outside the facility. A picnic on the hospital lawn or cookout in a nearby park can be quite a festive event, and may have the added bonus of stimulating the appetites of finicky eaters. A mere walk around the block for a long-term convalescent patient can easily be the highlight of that person's day. For many long-term patients preparing to return to their homes and schools, a few practice outings to the movies or shopping with a child life worker can help their readjustment. These outings are particularly important for children who will return to their community with a noticeable disability, since they offer children a chance to experience the reactions of people outside the hospital to their condition and permit the children to discuss their feelings with a trusted friend.

PLAY IN OTHER HOSPITAL DEPARTMENTS

Pediatric inpatients are not the only children served by a hospital. Outpatient clinics frequently exist within a hospital and are visited daily by dozens of children, as are the emergency room, laboratory, and X-ray departments. These children may not require hospitalization, but they are still in need of child life intervention to provide play experiences while they are waiting, to help them cope with feelings provoked by the medical setting, and to offer an interpretation of that setting.

The design of playrooms within these areas should follow the same basic criteria previously discussed. The area must be accessible by wheelchair, free of safety hazards, and should offer a choice of activities. Space may be limited, so the play area must combine elements attractive to various age-groups. In determining the specific design of each area, the child life staff must analyze the available space and the nature of the population served, e.g. will more toddlers visit the area than school-age children? Are the majority of the children receiving services themselves or are they waiting for others? What is the average length of stay? These considerations serve as guides in the allocation of space and the selection of materials.

The nature of the service offered in a given hospital department has a direct influence on the form child life activities take in that setting. The isolated crises of the emergency room call for swift, short-term intervention, while the regularity of visits to the outpatient department permits the development of on-going programming beneficial to parents and children. A discussion of the format and goals of child life programming in different hospital settings follows.

Pediatric Outpatient Clinic

The child visiting an outpatient clinic is spared the necessity of dealing with many of the most terrifying elements confronting the hospitalized child. Separation from parents is minimal, and the major adjustments of lifestyle which accompany an inpatient hospital stay are avoided. The entire experience lasts, at most, a few hours rather than days. Despite these advantages, an outpatient hospital visit remains a difficult experience for many children. The sight of unfamiliar medical apparatus may frighten them. The sound of another child crying in an examination room may unleash a stream of fantasies about the nature of this visit.

A principal goal of child life programming in an outpatient setting is to manage these concerns. The child life worker serves as an interpreter of the environment, explaining all that is unfamiliar and new. Parents alone may be unable to perform this task adequately, prevented by their lack of medical knowledge or by their own discomfort with the question asked. A parent may ignore a child's question concerning cries from the examination area, feeling that an honest answer may upset the child. Quite the contrary is true. The child may think that the unstated answer to the query is so frightening that even an adult will not discuss it. In such moments the child life worker may intervene and discuss, in a reassuring manner, the feelings people sometimes have when visiting a doctor. The parent observing this model of interaction is better prepared to deal with similar situations in the future.

As is the case with hospitalized children, many of those visiting the outpatient clinic will be unable to verbalize their fears and concerns. An ample supply of play materials can assist children in the expression of their feelings. Art materials of various sorts, puppets, dolls, and medical paraphernalia are excellent tools for eliciting the often hidden discomforts of children in the medical environment. The child life worker who discovers such concerns may, in many cases, correct misconceptions or offer reassurance. Children may need to know that their parents can remain with them in the examination room or that they are not seeing the doctor because they have been bad.

Insights culled from a child's play provide valuable information for other staff members. Therefore it is important that the child life worker maintain open communications with other medical personnel. Needless trauma to the child and frustration for the staff can often be avoided when simple observations from the play area are shared. A child may request, for example, that instruments to be used on her be first "tested" on her teddy bear. Complying with this wish is an easy matter, provided the staff is aware of it. Another child may reveal a fear of mutilation of his body. A doctor who knows of this fear can reassure the child that his body is not being harmed by the examination.

The play of children in outpatient clinics may have implications beyond the immediate response to the medical environment. The activities of some children may reveal a delay in their development. An observation such as this is particularly important for young children under school age. Their periodic visits to the clinic may be the only contact these children will have with child development professionals until they enter school. As a result of the child life worker's observations, children may be tested further and their parents advised of appropriate programming to assist the child.

The child life worker in an outpatient setting is in an excellent position to observe the interactions of children and parents, noting how they communicate, play together, and how the parent deals with management of the child's behavior. Occasionally the child life worker may detect signs of severe strain in the relationship, characterized by a lack of parental interest in the child, hostile verbal commands, or disciplining of the child through physical force. A description of this behavior must be communicated to other involved professionals, for it may serve as a warning of potential child abuse.

In addition to observing the interaction of parent and child, the child life worker should initiate means of improving the relationship. Many parents simply do not know how to play with their children, and they often welcome an opportunity to learn the skill. The child life worker can offer informal instruction, modelling, and encouragement in this area, and can structure projects on which parent and child may work together. Simple instructions for these activities can be given to the parent to encourage their repetition at home.

Similarly, parents may be locked into a particular style of disciplining their children for lack of knowledge of acceptable alternatives. The child life worker models behavior management skills in the play area, thereby permitting parents to observe techniques for dealing with their children. The child life worker's actions may further serve as a source of informal discussion of the subject with parents.

Parent education in the outpatient setting may take other forms. Bulletin boards and pamphlets provide information on subjects such as nutrition, safety, dental care, and a variety of health-related subjects. Videotapes, films, and filmstrips can also supply essential information. The child life department and other professionals may also wish to establish special groups for parents. Coffee hours, parent support groups, or talks on subjects of interest to parents may be instituted, depending on the needs of the population served.

Some pediatric outpatient clinics have established more formal parent education programs in the play area. Morris (1974) describes a program at the Mount Sinai Hospital Pediatric Clinic in New York City, designed to promote the cognitive development and language skills of disadvantaged young children. The object of this program is to train parents in play techniques so that they will encourage and stimulate their child's play at home, providing appropriate developmental activities. Over the course of six months, parents participating in the program learned 12 exercises, each of which the parent would practice at home with the child until the skill was mastered. Beyond the individual exercises, parents learned the more important lesson that children need play in order to learn and that the efforts of parents can enhance this educational process.

Azarnoff (1970) noted that the basic goals of a play program in the outpatient clinic are "to make it easier for the child and his family to come to the clinic and to create an atmosphere in which the child is trusting enough to be cooperative (p. 218)." By providing play and reassurance for children, as well as information and support for parents, the outpatient child life programs create such an environment.

Emergency Room

The hospital emergency room presents a particular challenge to the child life department. By its very nature the emergency room is an intense environment, likely to display distressing sights and sounds to those who visit it. Children who must sit in the waiting area, either for their own treatment or for that of a patient they have accompanied to the hospital, must be afforded a way of coping with the experience.

A trip to the emergency room is a fundamentally different event for children than a visit to the outpatient department or most hospitalizations. In the latter cases sufficient time usually exists to prepare children for forthcoming experiences, while the time between the sudden onset of an illness or the occurrence of an accident and arrival at the emergency room is often inadequate for meaningful explanation. Attempts to prepare the child in the midst of a crisis will meet with little success.

It is also likely that the child's major source of support, the parents, will be under such stress due to the emergency that they will be of little support to the child. Anxiety in parents can only increase that existing in the child. If children suffer an accident outside the home or become ill while at school, parents may not be able to accompany them to the hospital, thus depriving children of even minimal parental support.

Many children found in emergency room waiting areas are not there for treatment, but were brought to the hospital by parents who were unable to find someone to stay with them at home. Frequently these children are left by themselves in the waiting area while parents accompany another child to an examination room. These unattended children must cope with the oddities of the emergency room on their own.

The child life program in the emergency room attempts to alleviate the concerns and anxieties of children and parents during the crisis situation. The presence of a play area in the ER helps defuse the intensity of the atmosphere by allowing the children to play normally, rather than sit in unnatural silence. The sounds of children playing can have positive effects on the staff, who may have accepted the solemn, nervous environment as unalterable. After the institution of an emergency room child life program in one hospital, an obviously pleased head nurse commented, "That's the first time I've ever heard children laughing in here!"

Children who are well enough can play while waiting to see the doctor. Resnick and Hergenroeder (1975), who studied the reactions of children receiving treatment at the Pediatric Trauma Center at Johns Hopkins Hospital, found that drawing materials and puppets were especially popular for emergency room play. These provided children with a vehicle for self-expression and were often diversional during painful or stressful periods. The authors noted, for example, that some children continued to draw, even when receiving treatment.

Other children who cannot play may still enjoy a visit from the child life worker who can greet them with a puppet, answer questions, and offer reassurance. A calm explanation of events from the child life worker can dispel many of the child's fantasies.

Children not waiting to receive treatment may continue to play uninterrupted in the reassuring presence of the child life worker. Through their play activities these children can reassert control over their environment, reveal their concerns and obtain important information about the confusing events.

Parents, of course, can be of immeasurable help to children in coping with an emergency situation, but frequently their own discomfort impedes the effectives of their support. Resnick and Hergenroeder noted that many of the parents they observed behaved in inappropriate ways, shouting at their children in attempts to quiet them or pressing the point of a moral lesson derived from the child's injury ("If only you had listened to me, this wouldn't have happened!"). While the parent's admonition may be true, such a lesson is not helpful to the child in the emergency room and only serves to reinforce any notion the child may have that medical treatment is a punishment.

Other parents, particularly those whose negligence, however minimal, contributed to the accident or illness, may be overwhelmed by guilt. Preoccupation with their blame makes them less available to offer their children necessary support.

In all of these types of reactions, parents need support from the child life staff and other professionals if they, in turn, are to offer their children the support of which they are capable. Giving the parent a role or function can refocus the energy they presently expend on guilt or anger toward constructive assistance of their child. By providing a book for the parent to read to the child or suggesting any other activity they can engage in together, the child life worker provides the parent with a role incompatible with the less helpful behavior.

Nowhere in the hospital is the need for child life intervention more acute than in the emergency room. Unfortunately, few child life programs have extended service to this area. As Resnick and Hergenroeder note, this situation is particularly lamentable since a visit to the emergency room is a more common part of the childhood experience than actual inpatient hospitalization.

X-Ray, Laboratory, and Other Waiting Areas

For many children all of the most dreaded aspects of hospitalization or medical care in general are encapsulated in injections or blood drawing. Pain is experienced, parents are sometimes barred from the scene, and, from the perspective of the unprepared child, the event may seem like an unwarranted attack or punishment.

The same is true of an X-ray examination. Although X-rays are "painless," the child who is asked to lie unclothed under a massive metal contraption and drink a chalky liquid may be justifiably frightened.

Children visiting the laboratory or X-ray departments need the same elements required by other children throughout the hospital to face new experiences with maximum emotional strength: (1) *play* to express their feelings and regain a sense of mastery, (2) *parents* who provide a feeling of security, and (3) *preparation* for upcoming events. The extension of child life services to the laboratory and X-ray waiting rooms assists the child in obtaining these essential elements.

Through play experiences prior to the procedure, the child life worker can assess the child's level of understanding and can provide accurate information when misconceptions are uncovered. It is common for children to fantasize about blood drawing or X-rays, conjuring fears far worse than reality. Aside from the common belief that these procedures represent a punishment, children will express other fears. Young children have a poor concept of anatomy and physiology and may fear that a needle stick will leave a permanent hole in their skin or that all of their blood is removed during a bloodtest. Others, knowing that an X-ray can "see inside of them," may worry that their innermost secrets will be revealed. The child life worker who discovers and dispels these fantasies, replacing them with accurate information, removes a major source of resistance to the procedures.

Whenever possible, parents should remain with their children during the procedure. For children under five years of age, the separation from parents may be more terrifying than the procedure itself. The fear of blood drawing, for example, is compounded when children are wrenched away from their parents and taken to a small cubicle, where strangers restrain them while the blood sample is withdrawn. How much less traumatic the procedure can be for children if allowed to sit securely on a parent's lap.

As the studies of Skipper and Leonard (1968) show, parents who receive greater information about a child's condition respond with less anxiety, which, in turn, reduces the stress in the child. Child life workers in waiting areas throughout the hospital should adapt these findings to their particular areas, providing information about procedures performed by medical personnel in their department. In addition to verbal explanations and bulletin board displays, the child life staff can develop a series of pamphlets offering simple explanations about equipment and procedures. Suggestions of ways in which parents can help their children during these procedures should be included in this literature.

The extension of full-time child life services to departments which do not serve a large volume of children may be impractical, yet several measures can be taken to see that many children receive child life support during the time prior to these often traumatic procedures. As mentioned earlier, an inpatient child life worker can spend time in these departments during their busiest hours. As an alternative solution, an inpatient child life worker, child life trainee, or trained volunteer could accompany children from the pediatric unit to the designated area. This option unfortunately precludes the extension of services to outpatient visitors. A final possibility would be to have trained volunteers, under the supervision of child life staff, remain in the waiting areas to offer services to children and their parents.

Sibling Play Area

The needs of the nonhospitalized siblings must not be overlooked in the implementation of the play program. As discussed in Chapter 3, the brothers and sisters of hospitalized children need to participate in the child's life in the hospital. Interaction among siblings helps maintain an intact family unit, prevents unnecessary worries in the children at home, and minimizes the separation of nonhospitalized children from the parents. To encourage the presence of siblings, yet not provide services for them while visiting, is contradictory. Siblings may be included in inpatient play activities, utilize the outpatient play area, or play for periods of time in a sibling play area.

A separate sibling play area serves several functions. First, it stands as visible proof to the parents of the hospital's commitment to the well-being of the entire family. Second, it provides a special play for siblings, who so often feel that they are neglected during a hospitalization experience. Finally, it allows the child life staff to deal directly with those concerns unique to the siblings of hospitalized children.

Summary

The only children who cannot be found playing during the waking hours of the day are those who are too ill to do so (a rarity!) or those who are severely upset. This is a fortunate condition, for the benefits of play to a child are many. In addition to enhancing growth and learning, play has the marvelous capacity to return power to children in essentially powerless situations. Since children in hospitals continually confront situations in which they are deprived of power and control, it is imperative that the child life department provide children with the opportunity for play wherever they may go.

CHAPTER 6

PREPARING CHILDREN
FOR MEDICAL ENCOUNTERS

BRIAN VISITS THE HOSPITAL

W hen four-year-old Brian approached the front door of the hospital, he leaped onto the black rubber doormat and watched intently as the glass doors slid apart. Before his parents caught up with him, Brian had opened and closed the doors several more times. Brian had learned this trick on his previous visit to the hospital, when he had toured the building. That day he had played with doctor equipment, watched a movie about the hospital, and seen the kind of room where he and his mother would stay. The man who showed him around the hospital let him try the controls on the bed, making it move up and down. The man also told him about the button that he could use if he needed a nurse any time of day or night.

But of all the things Brian saw on the preadmission tour, he especially liked that front door. Before the tour Brian had worried that once in the hospital he would never come home again. This thought continued to bother him throughout the tour and was relieved only when he was at last allowed to jump on the mat and leave the hospital with his parents in tow. Although Brian had learned a great deal about the hospital that morning, the most important lesson he learned was that children can go home from the hospital.

Brian had had other concerns since the day he heard the doctor tell his parents that he would have to have "tubes in his ears." The only tubes Brian had ever heard of were large and made of cardboard or metal. He felt that he must have done something terribly wrong for the doctor to want to stick tubes in his ears! Noting Brian's apprehension, the doctor gave him a reassuring explanation and showed him the type of tiny tube that would be used. The doctor reminded Brian of the many earaches he had recently suffered and told him that these tiny tubes would help stop that trouble. Brian felt better when he saw the size of the tubes and heard that they were to help him, but he still had questions.

Following the preadmission tour, Brian and his parents read the book about the hospital that the man who led the tour had given him. As Mother or Father read the text describing the sights, sounds, routines and personnel found in the hospital, Brian would repeatedly interrupt to ask for clarification on certain points. Inevitably after such sessions Brian would play with his own doctor set, recreating scenes he had witnessed at the hospital or had heard about from his hospital book.

By the day of his admission, Brian had learned a great deal about the hospital and its routines, as well as specific information about his own condition. Sensitive medical personnel involved in his care were cognizant of the child's need to know about the future and to express himself about the frightening aspects of the impending events. Brian entered the hospital with normal apprehension. The preparation and support given him were intended to help him cope with difficult situations he would undoubtedly face, not to disguise the reality of the circumstances, since it is easier for children to deal with fears if they are anticipated and their nature understood.

Brian's entry to the hospital stands in sharp contrast to a scene so prevalent in past years and not entirely eliminated today. Terrified children were taken to the hospital with no words of explanation, leaving many to believe that they were being abandoned. Parents acted in this manner believing it unnecessary to upset their children by explaining events ahead of time. Other parents openly deceived their children, luring them to the hospital on the pretext of going to the park or grandmother's house. Parents obviously don't proceed in this way in a conscious effort to harm their children or add to the terror of hospitalization. They do so out of their lack of knowledge of the proper course to follow or because of discomfort heightened by the stressful events. Medical professionals must lead the way in helping parents and children prepare for their hospital experience.

Efforts to prepare Brian proceeded throughout his hospital stay, with continual explanations of his new environment by staff members, preparatory information on all procedures, and a more extensive explanation of major medical procedures and surgery. Even as Brian neared the moment of discharge, the staff continued to provide preparation, informing parent and child of permissible activities and of normal post-hospital physical responses.

Preparation for hospitalization, then, is a process, not an event. The process is set in motion when the physician informs the parents that their child must be hospitalized. Throughout the preadmission period and during the entire hospital stay, the process continues with explanations and support given to parents and children. The nature and implementation of the preparation process will be the focus of this chapter. Research relevant to preparation will be briefly reviewed, and basic issues, such as who should be prepared, how, and by whom, will be addressed. The preparation process for an anticipated hospitalization (such as Brian's) and for an unanticipated or emergency hospitalization will be examined in greater detail.

RESEARCH ON PREPARATION

The benefits of psychological preparation for hospitalization and medical procedures are undisputed. A considerable volume of research has indicated its value to parents and children during hospitalization, as well as upon discharge. Researchers in recent years have turned their attention to specific elements within the preparation process which appear to generate the most benefit. Through knowledge gained from these efforts, those professionals involved in the preparation process can make corresponding improvements in their techniques.

Research on the Benefits of Preparation

In their review of the literature, Vernon et al. (1965) noted that preparation efforts in the studies published at that time focused on three elements:

(1) imparting information to the child

(2) encouraging emotional expression, and

(3) establishing trusting relationships with the hospital staff.

Four studies examined by Vernon, et al. (Jackson, et al., 1953; Prugh, et al., 1953; Vaughan, 1957; and Weinick, 1958) "showed reasonably convincing findings to the effect that psychological preparation either reduces the incidence of post-hospital upset or increases the incidence of post-hospital benefit (p. 21)." Evidence concerning in-hospital reactions of children was inconclusive.

The studies of Skipper and Leonard (1968), which were discussed in Chapter 2, added significantly to our knowledge of preparation for the hospital experience. In field experiments, mothers of hospitalized children were given more information about the hospital setting than mothers in a control group. The experimental group mothers were also given an opportunity to express their thoughts and feelings concerning the stressful event. Not only did these mothers show less stress during and after the surgery of their children, but the children themselves demonstrated a lower level of stress than those of the control group. The mean levels of blood pressure, pulse rate, and temperature of the experimental group were also lower.

The findings of Skipper and Leonard are important for two reasons. First, the elements of preparation of children outlined by Vernon et al. (imparting information, encouraging expression, and developing trusting relationships) can be applied to parents, producing a reduction of distress in both children and parents. Secondly, the study indicates that the positive effects of preparation can be perceived in the hospital as well as upon discharge.

The preparation studies of Wolfer and Visintainer (1975) represent a synthesis of the knowledge obtained from prior research. Through what the researchers term "preparation and stress-point supportive care" parents and children were given information (on a level and via means appropriate to the child's age), urged to explore their feelings and, as a result of the process, developed a trusting relationship with an individual who could offer support at stressful points during the hospitalization. A control group received routine care, which, for that facility, did not include preoperative instruction.

The results of their research underscore the benefits of providing preparation and support to parents and children prior to surgery. The children of the experimental group demonstrated significantly lower upset and higher cooperation at designated stress points than did children in the control group. Physiological measures (heart rate, ease of fluid intake, and time to first voiding following surgery) were significantly better for the experimental than the control group of children. Post-hospital adjustment scores for the experimental group children were also significantly better. The anxiety ratings of parents in the control group further proved significantly lower than those of control group parents.

Research on Methods of Preparation

While Wolfer and Visintainer were establishing the effectiveness of a comprehensive program of preparation, other researchers were probing the individual elements of the process to answer questions such as the following: What sort of information should be provided? How should it be presented? What is the relative importance of presenting information versus providing emotional support?

Johnson, Kirchhoff, and Endress (1975) explored the question of the type of information provided to children concerning forthcoming events. Children who were to have casts removed were assigned to one of three groups: (1) the *sensation* group, which was to hear a recorded message describing the sights, sounds, and feelings they were likely to experience during the cast removal, (2) the *procedure* group, which heard a description of the process of a cast removal, and (3) the *no information* group, which heard neither message. The researchers hypothesized that the sensation group would fare better than the other groups, based on their belief that distress results from a discrepancy between that which is expected and the actual physical sensations experienced. Thus, by accurately describing the expected sensations to children, the discrepancy would be reduced.

The hypothesis of the researchers was supported. Ratings of observable behaviors indicating distress were significantly lower for the sensation group than for the no-information group. The procedural group fared better than the no-information group, but the difference was not significant. These findings indicate the importance of including accurate descriptions of the sensations a child is likely to feel in preparation for any procedure.

Melamed and Siegel (1975) examined the value of filmed modelling in enhancing the preparation procedure. Children hospitalized for tonsillectomies, hernia, or urinary-genital tract surgery were assigned to one of two groups. Children in the experimental group observed a 16-minute film depicting a hospitalized seven-year-old male as he encounters many events common to the hospital experience. Children in the control group saw a 12-minute nature film of comparable interest value. Subsequent to viewing the movie, children of both groups were prepared for surgery in a comprehensive manner by hospital personnel. It was felt that the children who had an opportunity to observe a role model's encounter with fearful aspects of hospitalization would respond to similar situations with lower stress than children who, though prepared, had not been exposed to this modelling behavior.

The researchers reported a significant reduction in fear arousal among the experimental group as opposed to the control group, both preoperatively (the night before surgery) and after discharge (three to four weeks later at a postsurgery examination). The control group also showed a greater increase in behavior problems upon return home than did children in the experimental group. Thus, the opportunity for children to observe modelling behavior through a hospital film, coupled with comprehensive preparation of parents and children, may enhance the preparation process.

In a recent study, Fassler (1979) attempted to examine the role of emotional support in preparation of children by dividing a group of children hospitalized for tonsillectomy and/or adenoidectomy into three groups. Children in the experimental group were read a story concerning a young girl's hospitalization, following which each child was asked a series of questions designed to elicit expression of fears and doubts. Misconceptions were corrected, and all questions were carefully and honestly answered. Each child in the experimental group was then allowed to play freely with a set of hospital dolls and equipment, during which time a researcher observed, asked questions to probe the child's understanding of hospital procedures, and corrected any misconceptions as they arose. Finally, each child was asked to draw a self-portrait, indicating the site of the upcoming surgery. Once again, misconceptions were corrected.

The children of Control Condition I received a comparable quantity and quality of emotional support; however, they were not encouraged to discuss their hospitalization. These children listened to a non-hospital story and then played with a set of knight figures. The session concluded after each child drew two pictures. Children of Control Condition II received no intervention prior to the administration of scales to measure anxiety.

Fassler found the combination of information plus emotional support to be the most effective in reducing anxiety. The measures of anxiety among the Experimental Condition children were significantly lower than among those children in Control Condition II (no information or emotional support). For one of the scales used by the researcher to detect anxiety (the Callahan Anxiety Pictures Test), the children of Control Condition I fared significantly better than those in Control Condition II, indicating that the emotional support alone was somewhat effective in reducing preoperative anxiety.

Guidelines Suggested by Research

Although existing research does not provide answers to all questions concerning preparation (some of which will be considered in the next section), the studies to date provide important basic guidelines:

(1) Both children and parents should be included in the preparation process

(2) Information should be provided to children at a level commensurate with their cognitive abilities

(3) Emphasis should be placed on the sensations a child is likely to experience

(4) Parents and children should be encouraged to express their emotions throughout the process

(5) The process should result in the development of a trusting relationship between those doing the preparation and the family.

(6) Parents and children should receive support throughout the stressful points of hospitalization from a figure in whom such trust is placed.

BASIC CONSIDERATIONS

When instituting a program of organized preparation for hospitalized children, a number of basic questions arise. Among them are: Who should be prepared? Who should prepare the children? When should children be prepared for hospitalization, procedures, and surgery? How should children be prepared? What materials should be used?

Who Should Be Prepared?

All children who are cognitively capable of understanding simple explanations of events and procedures should receive preparation. A lower age limit, beyond which preparation is ineffective has not been clearly established. Vernon et al. (1965) note that estimations by various authors of this lower age limit range from two to five years of age. The latter figure seems unreasonably high, as children of this age and younger are capable not only of understanding basic explanations, but also of expressing their feelings concerning medical procedures (Erickson, 1958). Furthermore, some child life professionals have routinely prepared children under age two—even infants—but their procedures have generally been limited to allowing children to handle medical equipment and showing children the appearance of persons in surgical garb.

Guidelines established by Petrillo and Sanger (1980) are helpful in determining the proper course of action in preparing young children for surgery. The authors state that toddlers should be told about surgery or treatment just before it is to occur, while more verbal toddlers can be told a day in advance or early in the same day if surgery is scheduled for a late hour. Thus, young children should receive explanations of future events, although the time between the explanation and event should decrease with age.

Parents, of course, should be partners in the preparation process, receiving explanations themselves and assisting in the preparation of their children. The preparation of parents is especially important when dealing with children three years of age and under. Efforts to prepare these children may not be totally successful, due to their limited language skills and ability to comprehend. Young children are, however, sensitive to the parents, reacting to mother or father's anxiety. By providing information and emotional support to parents, hospital personnel can reduce parental anxiety, thereby indirectly benefiting the children.

The preceding discussion presumes prior knowledge of an impending hospitalization, a luxury which parents and children are frequently denied. In the case of emergency admissions the preparation process should begin as quickly as possible, offering children explanations of events prior to or during their occurrence. This is not an optimal time for preparation and may be of limited value to parents and children. Under the circumstances it is especially important to offer thorough explanations of all that has occurred after the fact. Children and their parents may still possess fantasies concerning the hospitalization and illness, which may lead to further difficulties if unchecked. (A more comprehensive treatment of preparation under emergency circumstances follows later in this chapter.)

Who Should Prepare the Children?

If it is to be thorough and effective, the preparation process must, of necessity, involve a number of individuals from various disciplines. From the moment a physician decides to hospitalize a child, and throughout hospitalization, from admission through discharge, children and their parents need information and support. Questions and anxieties may arise at the doctor's office, the admitting desk, the playroom, or recovery room. Ideally, personnel throughout the hospital should be sensitive to the needs of parents and children to know what is going to happen and intervene at appropriate times.

A single individual, however, should be responsible for the major preparation of a given child and family. Through repeated contact with the designated individual, the child and family may more easily develop a relationship of trust, a condition important to provide effective support during stressful times. The member of the health care team conducting preparation sessions may be a child life worker, nurse, or other individual with adequate knowledge of medical procedures and a thorough understanding of child development and the emotional needs of hospitalized children and their families. If child life staff members are not responsible for the preparation of all children, they should work closely with others conducting formal preparation sessions, providing consultation on play techniques and effective approaches to transmitting information to children of various ages.

Some authors have suggested that parents are the most appropriate source of preparatory information. While there are advantages to the preparation of children by their parents, e.g. the parent's possession of the child's trust, sensitivity to the child's moods, and familiarity with the child's communication, the disadvantages are great. Most parents lack sufficient knowledge of the medical setting, personnel and procedures to prepare their children adequately. Even when they possess essential knowledge of the elements of hospitalization, many parents are prevented from effectively transmitting it to their children because of their own discomfort in broaching the subject or because they lack knowledge of the ways in which children learn. The child life worker or other individual responsible for the major preparation of the child must develop a good working relationship with the parents, welcoming them as partners in the process, while recognizing that parents themselves need parenting. In addition to information and support, parents should also be given a role by the person conducting the preparation sessions. As experts on their children and trusted figures in their children's eyes, parents can enhance the preparation process by providing valuable information and by reinforcing the material covered during preparation sessions.

Parents may initially be hesitant about participating in the preparation process or may resist attempts by others to important information to their child. Petrillo (1972) explains the source of much of this parental reluctance: "A common belief is that the child will be overwhelmed by anxiety (an indication of the parents' own reaction) which in turn will trigger anger against the parents or provoke unmanageable behavior (pp. 25–26)." As a way of responding to these legitimate concerns, Petrillo suggests stressing the individualized nature of the preparation process based on the child's developmental level, medical condition, and past responses to stressful conditions. Parents should also be aware of the hazards to which unprepared children are vulnerable as they face hospitalization without support or control. Ultimately, Petrillo notes, children will discover the true nature of their situation and, feeling deceived, will withdraw their trust from parents. The support of parents for the preparation process can generally be gained by thus delineating the positive, methodical nature of the process and by drawing a realistic picture of the undesirable consequences of its absence.

When Should Children Be Prepared for Medical Encounters?

Our knowledge of an optimum time for preparation is unfortunately limited. In her essay, "The Role of Bodily Illness in the Mental Life of Children," Anna Freud (1977) stated the following general rule concerning this matter:

> By deciding on the length of preparation time before an operation, two factors have to be taken into account. A preparation period which is too lengthy leaves too much room for the spreading out of id fantasies; where the interval between knowledge and performance of operation is too short, the ego has insufficient time for preparing its defenses (p. 76).

According to this principle, children prepared weeks in advance of hospitalization have ample time to supplement the details of their explanations with fantastic elaborations of their own creation. They are further afforded time to brood over the coming (and distorted) events. On the other hand, if preparation comes too late, children are robbed of the chance to process the material into a usable form in the attempt to achieve a state of inner preparedness.

The determination of what is "too early" or "too late" is the subject of some debate. Vernon et al. (1965) note that authors considering the subject vary in their recommendations of optimal preparation time for hospitalization from three weeks to a day or two prior to admission. In practice, the timetable for the preparation process is often modified by such factors as the amount of time between diagnosis and admission and the length of time between admission and surgery.

Robertson (1958) suggests that preparation for hospitalization begin no earlier than a week prior to admission. A number of hospitals have followed this principle, scheduling preadmission tours of the hospital within a week of the child's admission. The exact length of time prior to admission for such a tour can be moderately flexible and should vary with the age and maturity of the child. The magical thinking of preschoolers, for example, dictates that they tour the facility closer to their date of entry to minimize the counterproductive fantasies mentioned by Freud, while older school-age children and adolescents may begin the preparation process earlier.

Major preparation sessions, in which greater detail of the child's surgery or procedure is discussed, are generally deferred until the child enters the hospital. Most often the preparation by the child life worker or other member of the health care team occurs the afternoon or evening prior to the event. Should the child be admitted several days before surgery, the material to be covered can be subdivided into several preparation sessions.

How Should Children Be Prepared?

The exact form which the preparation process takes will vary with the personnel involved and with the nature of the situation. Quite obviously, preparation for a tonsillectomy anticipated a month in advance will vary significantly from that for an appendectomy performed on a child admitted with abdominal pain in the middle of the night. A detailed examination of preparation for anticipated and emergency admissions will be presented in the following section. In all cases, however, effective preparation should include the following elements:

FACILIATION OF EMOTIONAL EXPRESSION. The individual preparing the child must have an understanding of the child's state of mind. Through constant encouragement of self-expression, the child's prior knowledge, misconceptions, fears, and anger can be revealed.

INFORMATION. The child must receive information presented in an age-appropriate manner. Children should be active participants in the acquisition of information, handling equipment and objects whenever possible. Procedural information (how and why something is done) as well as sensory information (sensations the child is likely to experience) should be conveyed to the child.

EMOTIONAL SUPPORT. During stressful periods of hospitalization, e.g. during blood tests, before and after surgery, etc., children should receive support from the individual they have come to know through the major preparation sessions.

As stated previously, parents must be included in the preparation process, receiving information, support, and the opportunity for self-expression along with their children.

What Materials Should Be Used?

In recent years numerous materials have been produced which may be incorporated into the preparation process. The use of doctor equipment, play hospital furniture, books describing the hospital experience, charts, films and videotapes can, when properly used, increase the child's interest and understanding. These materials should, however, be viewed as a supplement to, rather than a substitute for, the preparation process. Merely allowing a child to read a book, play with a doctor kit, or view a film on the hospital is an inadequate form of preparation. Essential to the process is a caring, knowledgeable individual, whose presence can provide security and who is capable of responding to the fantasies and misconceptions which will no doubt arise.

It is not uncommon for children to display increased anxiety after viewing a preparation film or reading a book on the hospital. Fassler (1979) contends that this increase in anxiety under circumstances where the child receives information directly from preparation materials rather than from human interaction is due to a lack of emotional support accompanying the information. Fassler notes, for example, that children viewing the hospital modelling film in the Melamed and Siegal (1975) study showed a significant increase in anxiety as measured by the Palmar Sweat Index upon conclusion of the film. The anxiety of these children significantly decreased following a thorough preparation session by a member of the hospital staff. Fassler concludes that a style of preparation whereby children are given information devoid of emotional support and explanations may, in fact, be counterproductive, creating new fears and misconceptions.

Using Audiovisual Materials in Preparation

Recognizing the potential harm that can arise from misuse of films and videotapes, the producers of an excellent videotape preparation series (the Mister Rogers *Let's Talk about the Hospital* materials, produced by Family Communications of Pittsburgh, 1977) have provided a set of guidelines for proper use. Among their recommendations are the following:

(1) Children should view the materials in the presence of an adult who can correct misunderstandings or fantasies the children may have concerning hospitalization or treatment.

(2) Young children should view only those programs pertaining to their own medical condition. Otherwise, they may imagine that they will be subjected to unrelated procedures explained in the film or tape.

(3) The materials should be shown to individuals or small groups of children, thereby maximizing the attention given to each.

(4) A short talk should be given before and after the viewing. Children should be encouraged to ask questions.

(5) If a child becomes too upset or distracted during viewing of the materials and these feelings do not pass in a short time, the child should be asked if he or she would like to stop watching.

When using any of a number of films or videotapes produced commercially or by the hospital itself, these guidelines should be observed. All materials should be thoroughly screened by the child life staff to insure that the content is accurate and is presented in an honest, yet reassuring manner. Where a given hospital's practice differs from that portrayed on the screen, children should be advised of these differences. Hospital furniture, the uniforms of personnel, and the administration of procedures commonly vary with the setting. A discussion of these differences can stimulate questions relating to other topics covered by the presentation.

When used in conjunction with other forms of preparation by a sensitive and knowledgeable individual, films and videotapes can be of great benefit to the child facing hospitalization. As Melamed and Siegel (1975) have shown, the observation of filmed modelling of a child's encounters with hospital experiences helps children in their attempts to cope with their own hospitalization. Through audiovisual presentations children can observe a variety of settings and events common to hospital life in a relatively brief period of time. However, a serious problem inherent in media presentations of this sort is that they are essentially passive experiences. Active involvement, so necessary for the learning of young children, must come prior to or following the presentation. During the program the child sits passively. While valuable information can be conveyed in this manner, more actively involving materials must be considered for use in addition to or in place of films and videotapes.

Using Books in Preparation

If children are merely read to from a book, the experience is no more active than that of watching television. However, if children are allowed to snuggle close to a trusted figure, to interrupt, to interject, and to ask questions, the process becomes an increasingly active one. Parents, for example, may be given a book which, in story form, describes the experiences a child is likely to encounter in the hospital. By providing parents with material to discuss with their children, the hospital spares parents the discomfort of not knowing how to talk with their children about upcoming events.

Books have many advantages and disadvantages similar to those of audiovisual materials. Many of the major experiences common to the event of hospitalization can be presented in an attractive, well-organized manner. An unfortunate problem with many commercially produced materials is either that they are too general to be of much benefit to a child's specific situation, that they discuss materials unrelated to the child's condition (explaining a tonsillectomy to a child who will be admitted for a hernia repair), or that they are misleading. A brief review of children's books related to hospitalization will yield many instances of children smiling during injections, playing postoperatively with no apparent pain, or cheerfully waving as their parents leave. Such a portrayal is unrealistic and can only increase the upset of children when they respond in a different, yet normal, fashion. Anne Altshuler's booklet, *Books That Help Children Deal with a Hospital Experience* (1978), provides a valuable critical review of children's literature concerning the hospital experience, establishing guidelines for selection of appropriate materials.

A number of hospitals have developed preparation materials specifically suited to their individual setting. Such materials can be sent to a child's home prior to admission or may be distributed at the preadmission tour. Having been designed for a given hospital, books of this sort can minimize the discrepancy between that which the child anticipates and the actual experience. A variety of other books and pamphlets can be developed to enhance preparation for other common surgical and medical procedures, e.g., heart catheterization, cystoscopy, general X-ray examinations, etc. In all cases the child life staff should be involved in their production to insure that the materials are accurate, convey an honest picture of the child's anticipated experiences, and are presented in a manner conducive to the child's learning.

Using Charts and Models in Preparation

Plank (1971) and Petrillo and Sanger (1980) stress the importance of using body outlines during explanations of procedures to children. Plank observes that "children of all ages can talk more freely and understand more clearly when a drawing is used as an adjunct to an explanation (p. 19)." An assessment of the child's understanding of forthcoming events can easily be made by asking the child to mark the site of the surgery or procedure on the outline. Misconceptions thus revealed can be promptly corrected. The actual location can be indicated; an IV, catheter, dressing, or other visible change the child will notice following the procedure can be drawn in the appropriate place.

As Petrillo and Sanger (1980) note, older children and adolescents are capable of understanding the inside of the body and prefer a more scientific approach to preparation. Body outlines depicting internal physiology and models of organs and body systems should be used with this group to facilitate their interest and understanding.

Using Manipulable Materials in Preparation

An adolescent or adult who has never had his or her blood pressure measured will likely be able to understand a nurse's verbal explanation of the procedure, based on prior knowledge of stethoscopes, past observation of similar techniques, and the ability to conceptualize the situation described. How different it is for children with their limited experiences and minimal abilities to conceptualize the unfamiliar. Young children learn by doing. They handle objects, tip them over, pull them apart and reassemble them to learn about the unique properties of each. A purely verbal explanation of the blood pressure procedure is of little value. The child needs to manipulate the stethoscope and blood pressure cuff; to try them on a doll, stuffed animal, or willing human subject, in order to understand the process. Obviously the child will not understand the biological import of the diastolic and systolic readings, but that information is not relevant to one so young. The child needs to know how something will be done, why it will be done (to avoid misconceptions that the procedure is a punishment), and what it will feel like. This information can best be supplied through demonstration with concrete objects and by encouraging the child's active participation in the process.

Whenever practical, real medical equipment should be used in preparing children. Stethoscopes, otoscopes, syringes, tongue depressors, and other medical equipment lend an air of authenticity to the preparation session and allow children to deal with fantasies they may have concerning their use. Some children, intimidated by the actual equipment, may prefer to handle toy reproductions or miniaturizations of the apparatus. These surrogates should be available. The real equipment may be introduced as the discomfort of children subsides.

Through the use of dolls, demonstration of procedures can be performed in great detail and in a manner which maximizes the child's understanding. If the child is to wear a cast, for example, an actual cast may be applied to the doll. This process allows the child to understand the construction of a cast and affords first-hand knowledge of the sensations involved. Similarly, other procedures can be explained with the aid of the doll. IV's can be started, catheters inserted, and dressings applied—all with the active assistance of the child.

Models of hospital furniture may be incorporated in the preparation explanations. Not only do these additional props enrich the play atmosphere, they also facilitate understanding. It may be difficult for a child to follow a verbal explanation of the journey from hospital room to the operating suite to the recovery room and back to the hospital room. But by acting them out with a play hospital bed, operating table, and gurney, the child more readily comprehends the sequence of events.

All of the materials described above have an appropriate role in the preparation process. The mere use of these materials does not, however, insure a successful preparation. They must be employed by individuals knowledgeable of medical procedures and sensitive to the needs of individual children. The proper and effective application of these materials in preparing children for anticipated and unanticipated hospitalizations will be examined more closely in the following section.

PREPARATION FOR AN ANTICIPATED HOSPITALIZATION

Under ideal circumstances, the preparation process begins in the physician's office with the determination that a child must be admitted to the hospital. One hopes this determination is made at least a week prior to the child's scheduled admission. In addition to information on the child's medical condition, the need for hospitalization, and specifics of the procedures involved, the child's physician should supply parents with information concerning preparation of the child for the impending events. As Petrillo (1972) notes, by answering questions such as, "How much does your child know?" or "What do you plan to tell him or her?" parents reveal their receptivity to the preparation process. Reluctant parents may need the sensitive coaxing of the physician if they are to see the value of the preparation process. Those parents already convinced of the importance of preparation should receive verbal guidelines from the physician as well as printed materials, if they exist.

A system of communication between the physician's office and hospital personnel must be established so that the child life staff and others involved in the preadmission phase of the preparation process may act swiftly in a frequently limited period of time. Many hospitals mail a packet of materials to parents prior to the admission of their children. Included may be a storybook for parents to read with their children explaining common situations encountered in the hospital. With this information parents should be given guidelines concerning typical fears of children and means of offering reassurance. Parents should tell their children, for example, that hospitalization is of limited duration and that they will soon return home. Children should know that parents will be with them at the hospital and may stay overnight. Since many children view hospitalization as a punishment, parents should be alert to this fact, stressing the idea that the hospital is a place where people help children. An invitation for a preadmission tour should also be included in this packet.

As valuable as this information may be to many parents, it should not be allowed to stand alone. Lack of time, limited reading skills, or the stresses inherent in a preadmission period may prevent a parent from reading or making use of this material. Parents should be contacted individually by the child life worker. This contact may be in the form of a personal visit to the child's home. Klinzing and Klinzing (1977) report the success of experimental programs through which student nurses visited the homes of children prior to admission, talking with parents and children about the forthcoming hospital experience, and answering questions as they arose.

In many settings a more practical means of contacting parents prior to the child's admission is via the telephone. The child life worker making the call can assess the parents' feelings concerning the hospitalization and determine their receptivity to discussing the events with their children. The caller should further determine the child's level of understanding of the situation, offering parents advice in supplementing the information already provided. Parents should be reminded at this time of the importance of stressing key ideas, such as the return home and the continued presence of parents in the hospital. The invitation for a preadmission tour should be renewed during the telephone call.

Preadmission Orientation Tour

Children who attend a preadmission tour of the hospital have an opportunity to experience the unfamiliar environment in a small dose. They have a chance to confront many unaccustomed sights, sounds and smells, which will then be somewhat less foreign when the young visitor returns for admission. The child's nagging questions can be answered and certain fantasies can be dispelled. Specifically, a preadmission visit is important to children because of the following elements:

FAMILIARIZATION WITH THE ENVIRONMENT. The shock of walking into a hospital merely for a visit is often great. The stress of accommodating oneself to new surroundings, while facing the further traumas of blood tests, X-rays, and encounters with numerous strangers, sometimes in the absence of parents, can be overwhelming for the child. Through a preadmission visit the child can begin adjustment to the strange setting and gain confidence as important areas such as bathrooms, playrooms, and nurses' stations are located.

FAMILIARITY WITH PERSONNEL. The child will meet a staggering number of new people during hospitalization. Through a preadmission tour the child has a chance to become acquainted with some of them and to learn the function of those with whom involvement will be greatest.

FAMILIARITY WITH EQUIPMENT. Instruments and apparatus which will be used in the care of the child should be introduced during the preadmission visit, with the child having an opportunity to handle and explore those that are safe.

QUESTIONS ANSWERED. The hospital visit may stimulate questions, which can be promptly answered in a sensitive manner.

A LOW THREAT EXPERIENCE. The child life worker or other individual conducting the tour should monitor the mood of the children throughout the visit. Children should not be forced to view areas or engage in activities against their will. It is more important that children perceive that hospital personnel are sensitive to their needs than that they conform to a predetermined plan.

GOING HOME. Perhaps most importantly, the child visiting the hospital prior to admission is allowed to return home, thereby dispelling fantasies that, once inside, children never leave.

Parents attending the tour also benefit by receiving additional information about the facility and services, by having their questions answered, and by themselves becoming more accustomed to the hospital environment.

It is most advantageous if the preadmission tours can be given for individuals or small groups. This arrangement allows parents and child to visit the hospital at their convenience. Greater individualization is permitted when the tour involves one or two children, rather than a large group. Areas of the hospital important to each specific child can be visited, and the particular equipment to be used with each child introduced. If, for example, a given child will require a urinary catheter following surgery, this apparatus may be shown without fear of unnecessarily worrying a number of other children who will not need it. Individualization further permits closer monitoring of the child's anxiety during the tour and is more conducive to the successful encouragement of questions.

In contrast, a number of hospitals, particularly those serving large numbers of children, schedule preadmission tours for groups at predetermined times. Johnson (1974) describes one such program developed at Children's Hospital National Medical Center in Washington, D.C. The program consists of a puppet show, tour, and discussion with hospital personnel. Through the puppet show children and their parents gain a realistic view of the hospital. The subjects of fear, pain, anesthesia, and the experience in the recovery room are discussed by the puppets and a nurse, who serves as a mediator between puppets and children.

By viewing the puppet show with their children, parents gain an understanding of information concerning the hospital which they may later reinforce at home. Following the puppet show, child life workers and nurses conduct a tour of the hospital. Children and their families are grouped according to the age of the prospective patients, with the younger children receiving a shortened version of the tour. Among the areas visited are the X-ray department, laboratory, parents' waiting room, the operating room playroom, the induction and recovery areas, and a nursing unit, where a patient room, treatment room, and playroom are seen. Throughout the tour children are encouraged to participate actively, handling equipment demonstrated, riding in wheelchairs, and turning the crank on a hospital bed.

Individual hospitals may vary the format of the preadmission tour. In some instances a skit portraying hospital routines, a hospital preparation movie or filmstrip is substituted for the puppet show. In other settings the group activity consists of an informal party where families may meet members of the hospital staff.

Hospitals conducting preadmission tours for large groups of children may consider showing the visitors a mock-up of a patient room containing all essential equipment instead of actually touring a pediatric nursing unit. While a child life worker and a single family may unobtrusively slip into the pediatric unit and locate an empty room for demonstration purposes, the entrance of a large group will scarcely go unnoticed. The natural curiosity of visitors to the unit will lead them to poke heads into patient rooms or stare at children attached to unfamiliar machinery, making patients feel as though they are on display. A tour of the pediatric facility can be an extremely important experience for prospective patients, but the visit should not occur at the expense of those already admitted.

A valuable component of any type of preadmission tour is a play session for children. Confrontation with the unfamiliar and often threatening hospital environment will undoubtedly increase the anxiety level among many young visitors. In the play setting these children can express their fears and reassert their mastery over the environment. The availability of medical play materials allows children to satisfy curiosities aroused during the tour. As the event of hospital admission becomes more real in the minds of children, the desire to "try on" the roles of medical personnel increases. Vigorous medical play inevitably follows the introduction to the hospital.

Of course, some children will avoid the use of medical play materials, finding this equipment too threatening at the moment. In addition to doctor materials, the child life staff should provide a variety of other play media. Materials which encourage emotional expression, e.g. drawing materials, clay, pounding boards, other dramatic play props, etc., will be especially valuable as children attempt to manage their anxieties.

By observing the play of children during a preadmission play session, the child life staff can evaluate the preparedness of children for hospitalization. Those children displaying unusually great anxiety may be observed more closely upon admission to the hospital. Concerns expressed by children during the preadmission play serve as guides for the major preparation sessions of children upon admission. At one such play session, a five-year-old boy scheduled for kidney surgery continually asked about the use of a urinary catheter, which he knew he would have postoperatively. The child life worker observing this behavior offered reassuring explanations, and transmitted the observations to the nurse who would prepare the child for surgery. The nurse was therefore alert to possible fantasies the child might have related to the catheter and was prepared to present an effective explanation of its function.

Before departing, parents and children can be given further materials to continue the preparation process at home. If no preadmission booklets were previously sent to the child's home, they should be offered at this time. The importance of discussing the prospect of hospitalization with their children should be reemphasized for parents. Bolstered by the encouragement and clarifications offered by the hospital staff, parents may approach the task with a new sense of confidence.

Admission to the Hospital

The research of Wolfer and Visintainer (1975) demonstrated the effectiveness of support extended by a trusted individual to parent and child during stressful periods of hospitalization. If preparation efforts have been conscientiously coordinated, the development of a trusting relationship can be well advanced by the time a child arrives for admission. The same individual who made the primary telephone contact with parents and subsequently met the child and family for the preadmission tour should greet them again upon arrival at the hospital. The presence of a familiar support figure can cushion the shock of a hospital admission.

The primary support figure can show the child to his or her room and offer a further orientation to the immediate surroundings. When the essential areas such as the playroom, kitchen, bathroom and nurses' station have been located, the child can be told what to expect in the coming hours. In addition to any information about blood tests, X-rays, or physical examinations which may be scheduled, the child and family should be familiarized with hospital routines, such as when and how meals will be served. If any special programming is scheduled by the child life staff, the particulars should be provided.

Major Preparation Sessions

After children have been settled in their new surroundings, the child life worker or other member of the health care team designated to prepare the child may begin the major teaching sessions. The most comprehensive exposition of this aspect of the preparation process is given by Petrillo and Sanger in *Emotional Care of Hospitalized Children* (1980). The authors present in outline form a series of basic guidelines for working with children of various ages, stressing the importance of working with the parents of infants, providing simple, concrete explanations for preschoolers, and introducing explanations of a more technical nature as the child moves through the school-age years into adolescence.

In planning teaching sessions, Petrillo and Sanger urge health care personnel to adopt the following guidelines:

REVIEW GUIDELINES FOR WORKING WITH THE SPECIFIC AGE-GROUP. This helps determine an appropriate method of presenting information and serves as a reminder of the concerns most prelevant at each age.

CONSULT THE PHYSICIAN CONCERNING THE CHILD'S TREATMENT PLAN. By confirming the treatment plan with the physician, the hazards of transmitting inaccurate information are avoided.

REVIEW THE PARENTS' UNDERSTANDING OF THE CHILD'S CONDITION AND DETERMINE WHAT INFORMATION THEY HAVE TRANSMITTED TO THE CHILD.

DETERMINE WHETHER THE PARENTS WILL BE TAUGHT WITH THE CHILD

OR SEPARATELY. While noting the necessity for parents to receive accurate information concerning their child's condition and the potential value of their presence for teaching sessions, Petrillo and Sanger suggest that parents be excluded from the sessions if they are "obviously anxious or uncooperative (p. 68)."

DETERMINE APPROPRIATE METHOD OF EXPLANATIONS. Means of presentation, including teaching devices, are selected, based on knowledge of the child's age, condition, and emotional maturity.

GATHER ALL TEACHING AIDS TO BE USED IN THE SESSION. Among the materials suggested for use are body outlines, dolls, anesthesia masks, and models of medical equipment.

COVER THE MATERIAL IN TWO TO THREE SESSIONS. The authors suggest that several sessions be planned, even when time is limited, to allow children to assimilate the information and to avoid overwhelming them.

OUTLINE MATERIAL TO BE COVERED IN EACH SESSION.

Petrillo (1978) suggests that the first teaching session give children a basic understanding of the surgical procedure to be performed. Children should initially be questioned to determine their understanding of hospitalization and surgery. Accurate responses should be reinforced and misconceptions corrected. All children should be reassured that they are not to blame for their condition. Simple anatomical explanations should be given to the children, followed by a description of the treatment they will receive. A body outline and doll may be used for demonstration purposes, with the child manipulating the equipment involved. As a way of assessing the child's understanding of the material covered, simple questions should be asked. If the child is old enough, Petrillo suggests concluding the initial preparation session with needle play, during which the child may draw fluid into a syringe and practice giving injections on a doll.

Should the child require the use of special apparatus following surgery, such as a mist tent, respirator, or blow bottles, a second teaching session should be scheduled to introduce this equipment. During this session, the individual doing the preparation can briefly review the information previously covered and assess the child's comprehension.

Medical preparation and surgical routines constitute the subject matter of the final teaching session. The child is told about fasting, the use of "special soap," the trip to the operating room, the environment experienced prior to anesthesia, and the induction process. Care is taken to distinguish anesthesia from nighttime sleep to dispel the fear that the child will awaken during surgery. The immediate postoperative experience, including the recovery room, the presence of pain and its relief are discussed. Mention of the pre-op medication is usually reserved until the end of the teaching session to preclude anxiety from interfering with the child's understanding of other information. Immediately following an explanation of the pre-op injection, the child may be encouraged to engage in needle play.

On the day of surgery, Petrillo suggests reviewing forthcoming events with the child. If possible, the person who has conducted the teaching sessions should accompany the child to the operating room.

Guidelines for preparing children for specific procedures can be found in chapter 6 of Petrillo and Sanger (1980) and in *Pediatric Diagnostic Procedures* by Susan Droske and Sally Francis, published by John Wiley and Sons in 1981.)

The format of the major teaching sessions employed in the Wolfer and Visintainer (1975) study varies somewhat from that described by Petrillo and Sanger. The afternoon prior to surgery a research nurse explained in detail the events that would occur the following day. Information was transmitted to young children in story form. They were encouraged to perform the procedure on a doll while the nurse repeated the story. Older children also used the medical equipment and doll, but were provided with more technical information and the story form was omitted. In addition to procedural information and descriptions of sensations they were likely to experience, the research nurse helped the children identify and practice behaviors they could adopt at critical points. Children were told, for example, that a blood test was unavoidable, but that they could help minimize the time required for the test by holding very still. The children would then rehearse this behavior, selecting accompanying responses, such as crying, counting, or giving verbal orders, if they so desired.

Wolfer and Visintainer felt the identification of the child's role and the practicing of behaviors were "essential to increasing his [or her] feelings of control and involvement in the procedure (p. 248)." This format of preparation was adopted for the child's blood test, preoperative medication, and transport to surgery.

Child Life Involvement Following Major Preparation

Often the primary responsibility for conducting major preparation sessions lies with the nursing staff. Under such an arrangement the role of the child life worker shifts to support the efforts of that group. The child life staff, with its knowledge of child development, can assess the teaching methods and materials utilized by the nursing staff, providing suggestions for change when appropriate.

Perhaps more importantly, child life workers can provide follow-up teaching and reinforcement of the concepts presented in the major preparation sessions. Plank (1971) observes that, "as in the other phases of a child's growth, it is not enough to be told a fact once or twice; it has to be assimilated. To truly understanding something unknown and fearful, a child needs opportunities to come back to it in his [or her] own time (p. 14)." The playroom is an ideal setting for the preparatory education of children to continue. Information encountered during the teaching sessions that children find particularly threatening may be revealed through their play. Once the areas of concern are uncovered, the child life worker may provide additional explanation or reassurance as needed. As Plank further observes, "Because the play room is so remote from medical procedures, the children have often found it a safe place to show these fears and to open up for further talks and explanation (p. 14)."

Nursing may directly contact the child life staff requesting further assistance in the preparation of a child evidencing particular concerns over aspects of the coming events. Intense anxiety surrounding injections, for example, or fears generated by the prospect of anesthesia may be observed by the nurse preparing a given child. In such instances additional play with the child life worker may reveal fantasies provoking the child's feelings and assist the child in mastering the fear.

To truly be of help in reinforcing and supporting the information transmitted to children during the preparation sessions, the child life worker must, of course, maintain close communication with the nursing staff. One must have knowledge of the child's medical condition and scheduled treatment if questions and concerns are to be addressed meaningfully. Offering information that is contradictory to that presented in the major teaching sessions not only confuses children but can have devastating effects on their trust of hospital personnel. Daily report sessions with the nursing staff and careful attention to patient charts can minimize this problem, but any information about which the child life worker is not absolutely certain should be verified before presentation to children.

The Postsurgical Period

As thorough as a child's preparation may have been prior to surgery or treatment, the process does not end upon completion of the procedure. Surgery is, at best, a difficult experience for children. They need an opportunity to work through their feelings following this major event. Plank (1971) notes that adults frequently work through their postsurgical feelings by continually recounting the events. "Children," she observes, "have the same need but are less able to tell spontaneously about their experiences. They need the opportunity for repetition, in dramatic play and in words, to allow them to go over the events that troubled them (p. 23)."

By allowing children to play through events following surgery, the child life staff helps children to gain mastery over that which has occurred. Furthermore, play may reveal misconceptions which, if uncorrected, can leave the child with a belief that the procedure was a punishment or that it was unsuccessful. One child's postsurgical fears arose after overhearing the conversations of physicians concerning another patient in the recovery room. In his drowsy state, the child was convinced that their concern was directed toward him.

Older children, less likely to play through their feelings, can nevertheless be encouraged to express themselves through various activities. Petrillo and Sanger (1980) suggest encouraging children to write or telephone friends, to draw or paint about the experience, to make a scrapbook, or keep a diary recording events and feelings.

Through post-procedural play sessions the child life worker can discover the aspects of the experience which children found to be most disturbing. The language used for explanations, particular sensations encountered by the child, or elements of the physical environment may prove to be a source of anxiety overlooked by adults. Klinzing and Klinzing (1977) note that, "This information can then be used to revise the procedure and make it less threatening, or to prepare other children more adequately to cope with the procedure if it cannot be revised (p. 75)." Thus, while postoperative play helps the child readjust to normal life, it also serves as a monitor facilitating the continual refinement of the preparation process.

Preparation for Home

In addition to the normal medical advice given parents upon discharge concerning medications, treatments, and future appointments, parents should also receive guidance concerning their child's emotional state. While they should encourage their children to resume normal activities as quickly as possible, parents must also know that a brief period of readjustment at home is normal. Children may follow the movements of parents more closely or need additional reassurance at bedtime. By talking with their children about the hospital experiences and providing a chance for continued play at home, parents can foster the readjustment process.

Frequently children are discharged with limitations on their post-hospital activities. It is important that children understand the reasons for these restrictions to avoid misinterpretation of them as punishment. The child life worker should discuss possible activities with parent and child that are entertaining and fulfilling despite the child's limitations. These suggestions will be particularly helpful when the child must endure long periods of relative immobility, while in a body cast, for example.

The child fortunate to have been prepared for the experience of hospitalization in the manner outlined will likely have few problems upon return home. The information and support extended to children from the moment of the decision to hospitalize through discharge significantly reduces their fear. Many children, however, are denied access to the full preparation process, being admitted to the hospital directly from a physician's office or via the emergency room. Means of helping children under such circumstances will be explored in the following section.

PREPARATION FOR AN UNANTICIPATED HOSPITALIZATION

Mrs. Perez tried to reassure her hysterical daughter as she drove toward the emergency room. Six-year-old Tina had fallen from her bike, injuring her right arm. Tina's mother was certain it was broken. She tried as best she could to tell Tina what she could expect at the hospital. Her words were lost in the crescendo of cries from the terrified child.

Hasty attempts at preparation by anxious parents in the midst of a crisis will likely be of limited effectiveness for children. If children are calm enough to listen to an explanation, a few words of reassurance are appropriate to inform them that people at the hospital will be ready to provide help. When children are overly distraught, the parents' efforts are best spent in providing comfort and security.

Once in the emergency room or hospital (in the case of children admitted unexpectedly from a physician's office), parent and child can gain support from child life workers, nursing staff, or other hospital personnel. If the child must undergo an immediate procedure, such as an X-ray, the setting of a broken bone, casting, or the starting of an IV, the health care worker should remain with the child and parent in a supportive capacity. That individual can supply them with information about the procedure and can help engage the child in conversation or activity. Klinzing and Klinzing (1977) note that information given to the child during a procedure should emphasize the positive, telling the child how the efforts of medical personnel are helping. The authors emphasize the importance of maintaining some form of interaction with the child, rather than allowing periods of silence: "Silence communicates. In the medical emergency, silence communicates danger and causes fear and anxiety (p. 74)."

The format that the preparation process takes after the child is established in the hospital depends on the nature of the admission. In many cases children undergo immediate surgery, thus denying the time or conditions necessary for presurgical teaching. If time permits a cursory explanation prior to emergency surgery, Plank (1971) suggests the use of a poster or booklet containing pictures depicting procedures and events before and after surgery.

Otherwise, major efforts to help these children must come after their surgery. The fact that an operation has already occurred does not remove the necessity for a child to know what happened, how, and why. The child life worker or other person must plan a postoperative explanation similar in nature to that described for preoperative teaching.

Children suddenly admitted to the hospital because of the discovery of an abnormal medical condition, e.g. diabetes, leukemia, etc., are also in need of explanations of their new environment, procedures, and the nature of their disease. As in all cases, these children should be provided information about diagnostic tests, presented in an age-appropriate manner. Upon confirmation of a diagnosis, teaching sessions should be planned and implemented describing the nature of the illness and its treatment.

The design of these sessions also should parallel that of the presurgical explanations, reassuring children that they are not to blame, and offering information in a manner which actively involves them through the use of body outlines, dolls, and medical apparatus.

As with all children, those who are admitted to the hospital unexpectedly should be encouraged to play through and express their feelings concerning what were undoubtedly scary events. Unlike children who were able to attend a preadmission tour and receive preparation from their parents prior to surgery, children hospitalized unexpectedly have little knowledge of the foreign world into which they have been thrust, heightening the shock of entry. Children who have had a previous, pleasant experience in the hospital setting are less likely to have their apprehension concerning their physical condition compounded by fear of the medical setting.

Unfortunately, relatively few children have had an opportunity for benign contact with the hospital prior to an emergency admission. Some hospitals are attempting to change this situation by providing hospital tours for children in their community. The structure of these tours may be similar to preadmission tours, with the emphasis changed from an impending hospitalization to an explanation of services offered should the need ever arise. Familiarization with the emergency room is an essential part of such tours. In no case, however, should healthy children — school classes, scout troops, youth groups — be included in the preadmission orientation tour for prospective patients. Children who are scheduled for admission need close, individual attention that is impossible to give if one is conducting a tour for a group of healthy children.

Hospitals may adopt other means of acquainting healthy children with the medical setting. Child life workers, nurses, or trained volunteers can visit schools, talking with children about the role of the hospital in the community, demonstrating equipment, showing pictures of various areas and answering questions. Schools may further be enlisted to aid hospitals in the dissemination of materials to parents and children. Pamphlets informing parents of the importance of discussing hospitals with their children (including simple guidelines for initiating such talks) can help to minimize the future trauma of many.

Summary

It was once assumed that the emotional strife of children in hospitals and the psychological upset exhibited upon return home were inevitable. The suffering of children was considered an unpleasant, yet inextricable by-product of the healing process. While all of the anguish of children in hospitals cannot at present be eliminated, it lies within the capacities of hospital personnel to drastically minimize the negative effects. A comprehensive program of preparation and support for hospitalized children and their families is a major instrument in the attainment of this goal.

CHAPTER 7

ADVOCACY AND CONCERN FOR THE ENVIRONMENT

FROM THE CHILD'S POINT OF VIEW

The staff gathered around to nod in approval and offer profuse words of congratulations as the artist put the final touches on the new mural in the pediatric unit. With its circus motif, it was an impressive sight indeed! Clowns in multicolored costumes chased lions and elephants, while a daring high-wire duo performed unfazed overhead. Other performers displayed their juggling and sword-swallowing skills, as men with large muscles adjusted ropes securing the "big top." Surely, with all of its electrifying activity and splash of gaudy colors, this painting was exactly suited to lift the spirits of pediatric patients.

Two-year-old Adam, noting the crowd by the nurses' station, wondered what was causing the commotion. The tenacious child pushed his way through a forest of adult legs, finally reaching the wall. Staring straight ahead he saw nothing but a blank wall. Could this have been the source of grown-up fascination? Turning toward the group, he saw that they too had been staring straight ahead at the wall, but at *their* level. Adam adjusted his gaze upward. There, more than a foot overhead, he saw the painting, not as a whole as had the adults, but in details that were accessible to his view. He saw a human-like figure with a stark white face, stars for eyes and an exaggerated frown, running from an animal. To the left of this scene was a man plunging a knife into his mouth. A terrified Adam hastily withdrew to the safety of his own room, with its pastel walls covered with the get-well cards his grandma had sent.

It is difficult, if not impossible for adults to view the world through the eyes of a child. The memories of our own childhood are distant, and in many cases have been replaced by a more idealized view of the way it "should have been." In effect, we are all somewhat confused experts on the subject of childhood, having lived through the era ourselves. Although we may have been frightened by the sight of a circus clown as a child, belief in the universal adoration of clowns is so strong in adult society that we accept it as truth without question. Much of the environment to which we subject children is conditioned in the same manner, based on adult assumptions about the preferences of children, rather than their actual needs.

As the case history above illustrates, hospitals serving children are not immune to these errors. Walls are frequently decorated with cute "child print" designs, chosen to coincide with adult perceptions of children's tastes. Equally often (and mercifully so) such decorations are placed at a level well out of the view of passing toddlers. Entertainment in the form of books, movies, plays, and costumed visitors are similarly selected, having passed the adult standard of "what kids like." (For an excellent discussion of mistakes hospitals make in decorating pediatric units, see Carol Hardgrove's article in *Hospitals* [1980].)

The adult mind-set which deliberately augments the environment in inappropriate ways through misguided intentions, inadvertently permits the presence of psychologically damaging conditions through blindness to the child's point of view. To gain entrance to the pediatric unit, for example, children may have to walk past the coronary care unit, where they are exposed to the intense atmosphere accompanying critical illness. Prior to a blood test, a child may be asked to wait for excessive periods outside a treatment room, within earshot of the cries of other children. Even the mere presence of an unexplained closed door in a child's room can be a cause of fear easily overlooked by adults. Failure to examine the hospital environment through the eyes of a child allows countless hazards to the mental health of children to remain unaltered.

Most insidious among the environmental hazards produced through adult misperceptions are those which do harm to children in the name of helping them. For years visitation by parents was severely restricted in the stated belief that visitation is upsetting to children. In many hospitals sibling visitation is still prohibited, with the rationalization that the ban is necessary to prevent the spread of disease. Preparation programs are resisted in many quarters as producing unnecessary fear in children.

Often no more justification is given for the continuation of a given practice than the convenience it affords staff members. Parents are barred from treatment rooms because children are more "controllable" in their absence. Children must lie supine, an uncomfortable vulnerable position, during blood work, to ease the task for the blood drawer. Times for baths and dressing changes conform more readily to the staff's break schedule than to the child's play time.

If children are to emerge psychologically unharmed by the hospital experience, it is essential that the environment to which they are exposed be carefully and continually monitored, using an understanding of the perceptions of children and adolescents as a guide. Child life workers, with their knowledge of development, their close contact with individual patients, and their relationship with other staff members, are in the most advantageous position among hospital personnel to evaluate the environment, including all practices affecting children, advocating change as necessary. The role of the child life worker as an advocate for children and their families and as an evaluator of the hospital environment is the subject of the present chapter.

CHILD ADVOCACY

In 1969 the Joint Commission on the Mental Health of Children (1971) released a report calling for the organization of a national system of child advocacy to work for the implementation of change for the benefit of children. Although the system as visualized by the Commission never developed, the term child advocacy remains, and with it is an ever-increasing understanding of the necessity for securing the fundamental rights of children. For too long children have been treated as less than full citizens, often relegated to the role of society's chattel. Courts have sanctioned the rights of teachers to strike children. Thousands of children are abused annually. Shocking reports of parents "voluntarily" institutionalizing their children abound. Hundreds of thousands of children are injured every year in accidents related to unsafe toys and playground equipment. (See Michael B. Rothenburg's article, "Is There a National Conspiracy Against Children?" [no date] for a more complete treatment of this issue.)

While the majority of the child advocacy undertaken by child life workers will likely pertain directly to the hospital setting, it is important that they, as well as all individuals involved in the care of children, remain knowledgeable about issues affecting all aspects of children's lives. Change for the benefit of children cannot be effected unless those who are intimately involved with the well-being of children disclose areas where change is needed and fully support its implementation.

Local, state, and federal governments are becoming increasingly involved in the regulation and delivery of health care, and therefore a corresponding number of decisions made outside the hospital affect service within. Limitations on the addition of hospital personnel, for example, greatly handicap the expansion of a fledgling child life program. The closing of a government sponsored health clinic may reduce the availability of ambulatory care to a neighborhood, leading residents to neglect minor conditions until they become serious enough to require hospitalization. A governmental decision to aggressively promote preventative health care measures among lower socioeconomic groups (members of which are hospitalized in numbers disproprotionate to the entire population) might reduce the number of children requiring hospitalization.

Since the decisions of governmental bodies can have such a profound effect on the nature of health care, it is incumbent upon child life workers interested in the provision of optimum health care to children and their families to become involved in the decision-making process. All of the efforts made by child life personnel to improve the quality of a hospital stay cannot guarantee that a child will return home free of psychological upset. The obviously preferable situation is to avoid the child's hospitalization entirely. If many children in the community are unnecessarily hospitalized due to their lack of access to medical care, the child life worker who supports programming to correct this condition is providing as valuable a service to the mental health of children as any service that worker might offer in the hospital.

Specifically, the child life worker can organize fellow professionals, concerned parents, and other community members interested in the identified problem. Every issue should be thoroughly researched, with specific recommendations made to remedy the conditions. Rather than merely urging the health department, for example, to increase immunization among the preschool population of the community, a proposal for implementation of the project should be developed. Professionals interested in initiating change should arm themselves with the information necessary to promote their case and contact governmental officials capable of implementing the proposed action.

ADVOCACY WITHIN THE HOSPITAL

The role of advocate within the hospital is frequently thrust upon members of the child life department without their conscious knowledge or intent to be so involved. An angered parent complains to the child life worker that "We waited all morning for the doctor, and he never came!" Or a tearful child confides that "A lady from the lab called me a baby 'cause I cried when I got stuck." When confronted with such information the child life worker is compelled to intervene for the parent or child, seeking clarification of misunderstandings, facilitating communication, presenting their point of view to other professionals, and seeking solutions to problems uncovered. By doing so the child life worker adopts the role of advocate.

It is the unique function of child life workers in pediatric settings that enables them to serve so readily as a parent or child advocate. The child life staff is highly visible, frequently contacting children and informally interacting with parents. After a few such encounters under pleasant, nonthreatening circumstances, the family soon accepts the child life worker as a trusted, supportive figure. The child life worker's interest and skills in enhancing communication conveys a feeling to the child and family that their ideas, suggestions, and complaints are accepted and encouraged.

Child life personnel enjoy a further advantage by being members of the hospital staff, while not directly involved in the medical care of the child. Chief among complaints registered by child and parent are those concerning the child's medical treatment. Parents are disturbed by the attitude of certain doctors or nurses, question medical decisions, or express anger over the inadequacy of communication concerning the child's condition. Similarly, children react to insensitive treatment by the staff, or to the folly of certain hospital rules, complaining that "The doctor said it wouldn't hurt, but it did!" or wondering "Why do I have to take my pajama bottoms off for surgery if they are going to operate on just my throat?"

Assertive parents and children will have little difficulty directly expressing their concerns to the offending party; yet others, intimidated by medical personnel or emotionally weakened by the stress of hospitalization, will be unable to do so. These individuals may find it easier to discuss their feelings with the child life worker, who, though not a member of the medical staff, may be seen as a sympathetic hospital representative.

At other times the dissatisfaction of children and parents may be directed toward nonmedical concerns such as hospital regulations or the inadequacy of facilities: "Where are we supposed to eat when the coffee shop is closed?" "Why can't I be with my child in the recovery room?" "Why can't my mommy stay in the room with me?" These inquiries may also be addressed by the child life worker, who, in the eyes of parents and children may be able to supply answers or may transmit concerns to the appropriate official.

Frequently, no specific complaint will be made by parents or children; yet, the child life worker will, nevertheless, act in an advocacy role to correct a problem detected. If, for example, a child required to remain in traction for an extended period is placed in a room distant from the nurses' station and out of the view of passing traffic, a child life worker might seek a room change to a visibly accessible location to avoid the child's feeling isolated and abandoned. Or a child life worker, knowing the work schedule of a child's parents, might arrange for the scheduling of a care conference when both parents could more easily attend.

When confronted with a situation requiring intervention, revealed either by a parent or child's comment or by the child life worker's anticipation of a problem, the child life staff must formulate an appropriate response. Two general classes of advocacy exist:

(1) *case advocacy*, through which problems are handled on an individual basis, and

(2) *class advocacy*, through which a general change in rules or practices affecting children and parents as a group is sought.

Case Advocacy

Much of the advocacy done by child life workers is on behalf of individual children or parents. Problems often arise that are caused by a singular combination of variables such as the child's personal fantasies, the attitude of parents, the nature of the disease process, and the physical structure of the hospital. Due to the unique circumstances, a general alteration of hospital policies would have limited effect in remedying the situation. Therefore, hospital personnel must intervene as each problem presents itself.

For example, a child life worker talks with the obviously disturbed father of a patient the night before his daughter's surgery. The father, who has limited mental capacities, must sign a surgical consent form, but hesitates to do so. He has misunderstood a portion of the nurse's explanation of the operation, and now fears that his daughter will be subjected to a more extensive procedure than anticipated. Since he is reluctant to confront the nurse himself, the child life worker intercedes for the father, asking the nurse to repeat the explanation using simpler language.

A seemingly infinite number of situations will develop requiring advocacy by the child life worker limited to the individual case. Among the more prevalent types of case advocacy problems are the following:

Presenting a Child's Viewpoint to the Staff

Many of the beliefs and fantasies of children are widely held and easily anticipated. Preschoolers, for example, commonly view injections as punishment. Based on this knowledge, general procedures can be established to reduce the concerns of children, e.g. children can routinely be reassured that an injection is to help, rather than punish. At other times, however, the concerns of children are so personal and unique that they are not readily expected or discovered. The child life worker who, through a relationship with the child and family, becomes aware of such concerns must present that viewpoint to other members of the health care team if necessary changes in care are to be made, as the following example illustrates:

Lana, age six, was severely injured in an automobile accident, leaving her blind in the right eye and largely immobilized. Her fractured right leg required traction, and her tender neck, a brace. She was quite withdrawn and showed little response to her surroundings, except for her marked anxiety when anyone entered the room or when her bed was changed. Through play and conversation, Meg, the child life worker, quickly discovered the source of Lana's concern. The slightest touching of the weights on her traction caused Lana extreme pain, and she wished to keep vigilant guard over them. Her diminished sight and immobilized neck, however, greatly reduced her field of vision. When anyone entered the doorway (to the right of her bed) or tucked in the sheets out of Lana's view, she feared that the weights would be disturbed. Once the staff considered the problem from Lana's perspective, effective changes could be made. Her bed was angled to give her a view of the door, the staff talked to her about their movements while out of her view, and a mirror was positioned to increase her view of activity to her right. Her anxiety subsided quickly.

Presenting a Parent's Viewpoint to the Staff

Parents may have a legitimate concern about the treatment of their child that they are unable to convey successfully to the staff. In such cases the child life worker may serve as advocate for their position, enabling other staff members to understand better the parents' perspective. For example, the parents of a terminally ill child, who have watched their child suffer for months in a hopeless battle with the disease, may wish to take their child home to die, rather than have her submit to yet another operation recommended by the medical staff. At best the surgery will prolong the child's life, but may mean that she will spend her last days under heavy sedation in the hospital's intensive care unit. Although the parents have decided to forego the surgery and take their child home, they want to do so with the support and cooperation of the medical staff. A child life worker, aware of these wishes, might present this view to other professionals, seeking their assistance.

Resolving Personality Conflicts and Clarifying Misunderstandings

Conflicts between parents and staff can often be attributed to the stress inherent in the hospital environment. Parents, dismayed by the temporary disruption of their lives, or unnerved by the failure of medical personnel to produce a satisfactory diagnosis, are emotionally vulnerable. The stress of hospitalization can lead to the misunderstanding of communication with staff, hostile reactions and bitter relations. Staff members, who frequently operate under similarly stressful conditions, may, at times, fail to offer an adequate explanation to families or may respond to inquiries in a brusque manner. While problems of this nature may not be easily solved, child life workers aware of such conflicts may help the situation through several actions:

ACT AS AN INTERMEDIARY, UNCOVERING THE NATURE OF THE MIS-UNDERSTANDING. If parents merely mis-heard a statement, clarification by the staff member can prevent deterioration of the relationship. In cases of unresolvable conflict or the parents' complete loss of trust in a staff member, however, a reassignment of personnel may be necessary.

DISCUSS PARENTS' ACTIONS WITH THE STAFF. Behavior by parents that staff members find unusual or irritating may be understandable due to the family's cultural background, to exceptional pressure generated by their particular situation, or to their personal mechanisms for coping with stress. The child life worker cognizant of these special conditions should share this information with other members of the health care team. If the staff is aware of the motivation behind parents' behavior, they may be more tolerant of it.

ENCOURAGE EXPRESSION OF DISSATISFACTION. Parents may, at times, freely express their concerns and dissatisfactions to neutral parties such as child life workers, while never directly confronting the individuals involved. Hostility toward individual professionals can mount, damaging the sense of trust and cooperation so often necessary for the child's well-being. The child life worker's efforts in such situations should be to support the parents and encourage them to discuss their feelings with the person they view as the source of the problem.

Cal's parents grew increasingly suspicious of their pediatrician, fearing that she was withholding information concerning their son's condition. The assurances of staff members that all test results had been disclosed failed to satisfy the wary parents. Their confidence in and communication with the physician steadily declined as they continued to conceal their dissatisfaction. One day, after hearing the doctor's routine briefing on her son's condition, Cal's mother exploded, saying, "How can we believe you? You never tell us the truth anyway!" Surprised by the anger, the pediatrician probed the mother's feelings to discover the source of her discontent. Thereafter, the doctor made a point of thoroughly reviewing Cal's chart with both parents daily. With the proper encouragement and support from the child life staff, Cal's parents might have been able to confront the pediatrician sooner, thereby avoiding needless anxiety for themselves and the child.

Removing the Barrier of Inappropriate Regulations

Occasionally a hospital regulation which has validity in general application loses its meaning when applied in a specific situation. In another form of case advocacy, the child life worker may seek exemption from the regulation when its enforcement places a child or family under unnecessary hardship. For example, inadequacy of hospital facilities may force a limitation of certain services or priviledges, such as overnight accommodations or access to the anesthesia area or recovery room to families of children over a certain age. To apply this age standard to a severely retarded adolescent or to an adolescent who speaks no English defeats the goal of sensitive treatment for which the services were originally provided. Under these or similar circumstances the child life worker should be prepared to intervene on behalf of the family.

Whenever a regulation is encountered which appears unnecessary or inapplicable under a given set of conditions, one should question its overall validity. Is it, in fact, necessary to place *any* limits on parental access to the recovery room or anesthesia induction area? If the conditions originally necessitating the regulation have changed, or if present knowledge of the needs of hospitalized children and their families mandates a different approach, the rule should be altered or abolished. By working for this more comprehensive change, the child life worker turns from case advocacy to that which influences children and families as a whole, class advocacy.

Class Advocacy

Throughout the course of working with families the child life worker will undoubtedly detect patterns in their reactions that transcend the idiosyncrasies of isolated situations. Many children, for example, are observed to be highly upset when first arriving in the pediatric unit, or children frequently suffer nightmares when staying in a certain group of rooms. The basis of these problems may lie in the architecture of the building, the decor, the procedures children must follow, or the personal manner of staff members. By locating and eliminating the source of the problem, the child life worker can effectively reduce the potential for trauma for all who enter the hospital.

It is important for the child life worker to be aware of the hospital environment, evaluating the structural design, the available services, procedures, and regulations, advocating change when an undesirable condition is identified. Child life programming cannot function effectively in isolation. Although care within a pediatric unit may be sensitive and enlightened, and the play program may be comprehensive, if children and families are subjected to horrifying sights and emotionally damaging procedures elsewhere in the hospital, the value of child life programming may be limited. Time which could be better spent preparing children for surgery or assessing their understanding of their condition will be expended on the resolution of feelings generated by avoidable unpleasantness within the hospital.

Furthermore, since it may not be possible for the child life worker to personally contact every patient, there must be a certain amount of reliance on the environment to convey positive messages to hospitalized families. If the admission procedure is prompt and pleasant, if the surroundings are attractive, and if the child has ready access to play materials, the family will gain a sense of welcome and security, even if early child life contact is impossible.

Guidelines for Environmental Evaluation

Before commencing observation of the hospital environment to assess its possible psychosocial impact on children and their families, contact staff members in the area involved, explaining the purpose of your activities. Ask their opinion of the environment, requesting their ideas for change. Problems which an observer might miss during a relatively brief period might be illuminated by staff members who confront them daily. The often heavy demands of their work schedules prevent hospital personnel from making desired changes in the environment, and therefore they may welcome your presence. Furthermore, when personnel are involved in the process from the beginning, they are more likely to be receptive to proposed changes. Agree to discuss all findings and recommendations with the staff of each department observed upon completion of the investigation.

When visiting each area, select an unobtrusive spot with a clear view. Observation should last long enough to evaluate the environment from the perspective of toddlers and preschool children, school-age children, adolescents, and adults. Each area should be viewed when use is light and when it is heavy, for certain problems may become apparent only when larger groups are present. For example, the admitting area may seem pleasant and attractive, with short waits and ample activity for children and parents during certain periods, only to prove woefully inadequate, with scarce seating and excessive waiting at other times.

Observers should attempt to enter the mind of the child, reacting to the environment as a child encountering it for the first time. It is helpful to select children of a given age and closely follow their movements. Note how they respond. What attracts them? What repels them? Does the environment pique their curiosity or arouse their anxiety? What is responsible for these reactions? What can be done to enhance or diminish these responses?

When assessing the impact of the environment on various age-groups, it will be helpful to consider the following standards.

Toddlers and Preschoolers

The magical, animistic thinking of very young children leaves them vulnerable to many misperceptions of the environment. When in each setting be aware of those elements which are most likely to arouse frightening fantasies in the child's mind. Can unexplained noises be heard? Is medical apparatus in view? Do other children frequently emerge from a door crying? Can older, critically ill patients be seen?

The misperceptions of children may be compounded by their smallness of stature. View each setting from the preschooler's level to see what elements appear more frightening, or are more open to misperception, when viewed from that perspective. It is also important to note how the child's size affects adaptation to the environment. Is the furniture too large? Are toy shelves too high? What dangers exist on the child's level? Have they been effectively eliminated?

As well as being safe, nonthreatening and functional, the environment at the preschooler's level should be interesting and challenging. Children should have access to a variety of visual and tactile stimuli. Walls, rather than being blank at the child's level, should be decorated with colorful patterns, materials of differing textures, or with activity centers comprised of manipulable objects such as gears, wheels, and levers. Waiting areas should provide activities appropriate to the young child's interests.

Preschoolers are highly dependent on their parents. Every area should allow for the presence of parents and should encourage their interaction with their children. In waiting areas, for example, easily movable adult-sized chairs can be provided to enable parents to position themselves next to their child's activity. Instructions for simple activities can be available and directed toward parents, therby promoting the involvement of parents with their children.

Although dependent on parents, preschoolers are striving for a sense of autonomy, seeking constantly to assert a measure of independence. The environment throughout the hospital should facilitate the child's attempts at self help. Important areas such as restrooms should be clearly labelled with picture symbols for easy identification by prereaders. Safe toys should be accessible from low, shallow shelves. Eating areas should be designed to allow children to feed themselves with minimum worries about the difficulty of clean up.

School-Age Children

When evaluating environments used by children of this age, one must allow for their increased developmental capacities. School-age children are more sociable, capable of developing relationships with peers and adults outside their families. They display great intellectual curiosity, seeking explanations for phenomena observed. Skills acquired during earlier years, such as ambulation, verbalization, and the ability to care for oneself, are practiced in increasingly complex forms, offering a source of pride in accomplishment. Threats to the child's ability to exert control are resisted.

In light of these characteristics, hospital environments for school-age children should promote social interaction, provide for intellectual exploration, and permit the child the highest degree of control possible. Areas where children can gather, or where they are required to wait, should be large enough to allow several children to participate in a group activity. The presence of a table with appropriate-sized chairs and suitable activities, such as games, craft projects, or art materials, enhance the formation of groups. In addition to the provision of stimulating activities, hospital personnel can accommodate the intellectual curiosity of school-age children by the creation of educational displays and interest centers. Such materials can be used to provide explanations about health, the human body, or the function of various hospital departments. Lindheim et al. (1972), for example, suggest that, "An X-ray department waiting room might have posters showing how the machines work and supply discarded plates for children to examine."

While hospitalization necessarily removes much of the control so important to children, especially those of school age, the environment should allow opportunities for the child to exert mastery and demonstrate the ability to control. For example, doorways to bathrooms and patient rooms should be easily opened by children, to prevent the embarrassment of asking adults for assistance. Drinking fountains, sinks, and telephones should be placed at a level where children in wheelchairs have ready access. Activities should be available on a self-serve basis.

Some accommodations similar to those made for preschoolers should also be made for the school-age child. Obviously frightening stimuli should be kept out of the range of the children. Although school-age children are less consumed by fantasies than preschoolers, they are certainly not immune, and the viewing of critically ill patients or hearing the sounds of children in distress are disconcerting for anyone requiring medical attention. All areas should also be screened for the elimination of safety hazards, and accommodations for parents accompanying children to various areas of the hospital should be provided.

Adolescents

Of paramount concern for adolescents is the need for privacy and the opportunity to assert independence. Hospital environments serving adolescents should sensitively reflect these needs. Adolescents should be offered the opportunity to speak on their own behalf, rather than relying on parents to provide the information. For example, during the admission process questions can be directed toward the adolescent. The location of this admission interview should, however, be isolated in deference to the patient's concern for privacy in potentially embarrassing matters.

The provision of curtains around the adolescent's bed, personal space in the bedroom, and lockable bathroom doors provide security for patients concerned about their body image. By providing a separate adolescent lounge, which patients may decorate to suit their tastes, cooking facilities for preparing snacks, recreational opportunities, and access to friends via telephone and visits, the hospital promotes a patient's sense of independence and fosters important peer relationships.

Areas used by adolescents are frequently visited by younger patients as well. Although adolescents may have a living unit separate from younger children, all patients may be admitted to the hospital in a common area and may use the same corridors to reach departments such as radiology or the laboratory, which serve all ages. Because of the presence of younger children in these locations, hospital personnel often feel compelled to decorate hallways, waiting rooms, and other areas in a manner they feel appropriate for the more vulnerable preschool patients. "Child print" curtains are installed and storyboook murals cover the walls. The presence of such decor can create an uncomfortable and embarrassing experience for adolescent patients and conveys insensitivity on the part of the staff. Through the use of abstract designs, varying textures, and brightly colored patterns, interesting and attractive areas can be created which appeal to all ages and avoid branding the setting as the province of only a single age-group.

Parents

Even as the hospital environment may alternately arouse the interests of patients and convey a sense of belonging, or instill fear and provoke mistrust, so may the environment affect parents. Included in the evaluation of the hospital setting should be a survey of the tacit messages transmitted to parents through the architecture, furniture arrangement, decor, and procedures which affect them. As discussed in Chapter 3, parents in the hospital need guidance, support, and information if they are to function effectively and provide meaningful support to their children. The sensitive hospital environment can reinforce the efforts of hospital staff to meet the needs of parents. Hardgrove (1972) notes, for example, that the architecture of the pediatric unit can encourage parents to take advantage of rooming-in policies. The presence of a parents' work station, storage space, and food preparation facilities indicates to parents that a hospital's rooming-in policy is more than mere words on paper.

Hospital staff may make use of wall space to convey positive messages and information to parents. Signs should be phrased in a manner that indicates to parents that they are indeed welcomed as valued partners in the care of their children. Instead of the negatively worded "NO VISITING 10 PM to 8 AM, Except for Parents," a sign might read: "Parents, You Are Welcome 24 Hours! Others Visitors from 8 AM to 10 PM." The transmission of information via the walls may also help counter the stereotypes of hospital settings held by some parents. "Maps and charts on the wall can inform parents and encourage curiosity and questioning about the children in contrast to the secrecy so prevalent in most hospitals (Hardgrove, 1972, p. 56)." Bulletin board displays can inform parents of when the playroom and cafeteria are open, where to find nearby stores, inexpensive restaurants within walking distance, the names of health care workers on the unit, and other helpful information.

The arrangement of hospital furniture can serve to reassure parents that they retain their role as caretaker of their child and can facilitate the interaction between parent and child. The positioning of parent sleeping facilities next to the child, for example, indicates the importance of parents to their children and enables parents to more easily participate in their child's care. Similarly, the seating arrangement in waiting areas can allow parents and their children to mix freely and share a common activity.

An important part of the environment in any hospital area for parents and their children of any age is the interaction between staff and those visiting the setting. When observing in each area take note of the quality of this communication. Are families greeted promptly and courteously? Do staff members acknowledge the presence of children or do they mistakenly talk directly to parents about the children as if they were not present? If delays occur, are they explained satisfactorily? Are staff members sensitive to the anxiety of children and parents? As with any elements of the environment, if problems are discovered in staff/parent interaction, the child life worker should be prepared to act as an advocate for change. Policy alteration, staff workshops on communication, or the reassignment of personnel are among measures which may be employed to bring about effective change.

Areas of Special Importance

The potential for creating or exacerbating emotional distress in children and their parents due to environmental factors exists in all areas of the hospital, including such nonmedical areas as the playroom, gift shop, and snack bar. A thorough investigation of the hospital environment will include an evaluation of all these areas. It is especially important, however, to concentrate one's efforts on those areas of the hospital which, because of the amount of time children spend there or because of the stresses inherent in procedures performed there, represent the greatest potential for trauma. Among these areas are the entrances to the hospital, corridors, waiting areas, treatment rooms, patient rooms, and the nursing unit in general.

Entrance to the Hospital

Arrival at the hospital is a stressful time for children and their parents, even in nonemergency situations. Hospitalization, for many, is a new and threatening experience, bound to entail numerous moments of apprehension and uncertainty, as well as a measure of physical and emotional pain. The family pondering this imminent future may either have their most discomforting fears reinforced by their first visual contact with the hospital or may find unexpected comfort. Parents who have difficulty locating the pediatric entrance to the hospital and, once inside, are overwhelmed by a massive and chaotic lobby will readily perceive the hospital as an uncaring, impersonal institution. The foreboding nature of the lobby and the realization that parents, too, are anxious increase the vulnerability of the children.

When examining the entrance to the hospital, attempt to comprehend the feelings of children and parents approaching it for the first time. Determine which elements produce discomfort, assessing the changes that can be made to reduce these feelings. For example, it is impossible to alter the fortress-like external appearance of a large medical complex; yet it is quite possible to mark driveways and parking areas clearly to identify the appropriate entrance with minimum difficulty. A stark, concrete entrance can be made more appealing through landscaping or the construction of an outdoor play area.

Once inside the door, the family's initial impression of the hospital should be pleasant and should minimize feelings of personal confusion or disregard by the hospital. This can be accomplished through architectual alterations or through immediate contact by hospital personnel. If the lobby area is excessively large, perhaps a portion of it could be eliminated from view by partitions, creating a more intimate, cheerfully decorated admitting area. Part of the lobby space might be devoted to a play area that could serve children while they wait for admission and would immediately convey familiarity and acceptance to children.

If all patients, adult and pediatric, are admitted in a common area and it is impossible to satisfactorily redesign the area to make it more receptive to children and their families, then perhaps another entrance could be used for pediatric patients. Ideally, such an entrance should be located near the pediatric unit to avoid extended travel through hospital corridors.

In addition to architectural or design changes, the hospital entrance can be made more comprehensible and inviting by the presence of staff members who greet the family, orienting them to their new surroundings. A child life worker who has had previous contact with the family via the telephone and preadmission tour is an obvious choice for this role. As an alternative, a receptionist, knowledgeable of the needs of hospitalized children and their families, should be available to perform this function.

The importance of the preadmission tour is evident upon arrival of the family at the hospital. Those who have had an opportunity to participate in such a tour have previously confronted the peculiarities of the hospital setting, finding them more familiar, and therefore less troublesome, upon admission. Through a combination of preadmission tour activities and careful attention to the environment of the hospital entrance, the potential for trauma at the earliest stage of hospitalization is greatly reduced.

Admitting Procedures

Efforts to improve the environment of a hospital entrance may be quickly counteracted by the frustrations parents and children experience with admission procedures. Excessive delays, compounded by the absence of meaningful activities or interest centers for children and parents, present an inauspicious introduction to hospital routines. Hospitals seeking to minimize problems in the admission process may follow one of several possible approaches.

Patients scheduled for hospital admission may be given an appointment specifying their time of arrival at the hospital. By staggering admission appointments throughout the day, there is less chance that a large group of patients will appear at the same time, increasing the waiting period for many. Inevitably, some waiting time will occur. This time may be more tolerable if children are provided with suitable space and materials for play (a child life worker or volunteer may be assigned to this area during busy periods), and if displays or information of interest to parents is available.

As a preferable alternative, the period spent in the admitting area may be greatly reduced or eliminated. For example, the necessary forms may be given to a parent prior to admission, to be completed and returned upon arrival at the hospital or by mail. This procedure reduces the frequently lengthy interviewing process, shortening the child's wait. Lindheim et al. (1972) suggest delaying admitting procedures entirely until after children have been made comfortable in their rooms.

When evaluating the admission procedures of a hospital, be cognizant of the early demands placed upon the child. Are children given an opportunity to explore their new surroundings and become familiar with them, or are they immediately required to submit to medical procedures in the laboratory or X-ray department? It is disorienting and frightening for children to experience a succession of threatening situations before introduction to their own quarters in the pediatric unit. Such procedures should be delayed until children have had an opportunity to become accustomed to their new environment, discovering positive elements such as their personal space in the room and the activities of the playroom.

Corridors

The passageways that children and families must use to move from one area of the hospital to another present hazards to their emotional well-being that are frequently ignored. As Lindheim et al. (1972) note:

> Hospital circulation patterns are generally so complex, involving several changes of level and direction, that adults as well as children feel lost. Trips from the nursing unit to other hospital sections through hallways cluttered with strange equipment or lined with alarmingly ill patients can intensify the anxiety of a child headed for a new and possibly painful experience (p. 17).

While new hospitals might be designed to eliminate the seemingly endless corridors, placing support services such as the laboratory and X-ray department in close proximity to the pediatric unit, presently existing hospitals must seek other solutions. Among the suggestions made by Lindheim et al. for improving the environment of hallways are the following:

(1) Improve the decor of the corridors "by using warm colors and surfaces, by carpeting the floor, by using diffused lighting, by locating stops of interest along the way, and by opening the

perspective at intervals to interesting views (p. 17)."

(2) Provide storage areas off of corridors to eliminate the clutter and threatening appearance of equipment constantly in view.

(3) Provide waiting areas for the sicker patients off the hallway so they will not be in view of pediatric patients using the corridor.

When conducting the environmental evaluation, the child life worker may discover that children are required to make numerous trips to remote parts of the hospital that are simply unnecessary. For example, trips to the laboratory for routine blood drawing or to the EKG office for an electrocardiogram could be avoided if personnel from those departments visited children in the pediatric unit. By eliminating these treks to remote parts of the hospital, children have less exposure to the frequently confusing and frightening environments of hospital corridors.

In addition to advocating policy changes that reduce the traffic in hallways and offering ideas for redecoration, the child life worker can minimize the threat presented by corridors by conducting playful explorations of the areas with patients. School age children in particular enjoy the opportunity to investigate the environment beyond the pediatric unit, welcoming an expansion of their horizons—if a painful or frightening procedure does not await them at the end of the journey. Equipment or scenes which, when viewed without explanation, seem threatening, may be studied with interest when presented to children in an informative way by a trusted adult. By touring selected portions of the hospital in this manner, children become more accustomed to the previously confusing pathways, thereby making the entire hospital environment more comprehensible and less threatening.

Waiting Areas

Although a certain amount of time spent in the confines of hospital waiting areas is unavoidable, the frustrations of children, parents, and staff frequently resulting from such waits can be diminished. The discomfort arising from these periods is due, primarily, to their excessive length, the anxieties of the participants, and the lack of involving activities during the wait. When these elements are present in a waiting area, ameliorative measures should be promoted.

Mechanisms for reducing the amount of patient and parent time spent in waiting rooms should be explored. Prior to a scheduled event in another department, children should be allowed to remain "on call" in the familiar surroundings of their hospital unit until the department is ready for them. If unforeseen delays occur, patients may spend the excess time in the pediatric playroom or their own rooms, rather than a remote waiting area. When ready, personnel in the department can call for children, allowing enough time for their travel to the area.

In departments such as the emergency room or other areas where unscheduled procedures are often performed, the system described is obviously unworkable. The length of waiting periods in these areas is unpredictable and often excessive. It is essential, therefore, to provide a benign, stimulating environment during these times. As discussed previously, all waiting areas must be free of those factors that easily heighten the anxiety of patients. Medical equipment should be stored out of view. As Lindheim et al. (1972) have suggested, separate areas for more sick patients should be provided to avoid frightening waiting children and to insulate those patients from the curious stares of others. Treatment rooms should be located in an area which minimizes the amount of noise audible from the waiting area.

In addition to removing emotionally threatening stimuli, it is necessary to provide materials of interest to parents and children during waiting periods. Young children deprived of interesting play materials will search for substitute items with which to continue play. When their attention turns to climbing cabinets or fishing for lost coins between the cushions of chairs, the frustration of parents and staff increase. Merely providing a supply of play materials, with no guidance from child life supervision, may also prove inadequate. Pieces are easily lost, with parts left in disarray when a child is called for a procedure, leaving subsequent children with a pile of meaningless and perhaps dangerous rubble. If supervision cannot be provided in a given waiting area, a limited number of safe, durable items should be kept available. Older children, adolescents, and parents can be informed and entertained through slide-tape presentations, displays, and pamphlets on a variety of medical and nonmedical topics.

Treatment Rooms

The common vision of a treatment room contains sterile white walls, banked with ominous equipment surrounding a cold metal table. The nervous minutes spent in such a location while waiting for the nurse or doctor seem endless. As with other areas, the anxiety resulting from a visit to a treatment room can be reduced through procedureal and physical manipulations in the environment. Procedurally, children should not be introduced to the treatment room until the personnel to work with them are prepared to do so. These areas are totally unsuitable for prolonged waits, generally being of limited space and unsafe for even moderately active play. Recognizing, however, that emergency situations in a department may necessitate a longer wait in the treatment room than desirable, each area should be provided with quiet play materials such as books, puppets, crayons, and paper.

It is important to keep the amount of medical equipment visible in the treatment room at a minimal level. Preschool children with their egocentric view of the world will believe that all equipment present is intended for use on them. Thus, the more equipment in view, the more fantasies their minds will spin. By providing ample closet space, much of the equipment can easily be stored out of view, while remaining available for immediate use. Pieces which cannot be stored may be introduced to the child by staff members in an informative way, reassuring children, when appropriate, that the apparatus is not necessarily for their treatment.

Antiseptic white walls should be replaced with warmer, more cheerful colors. The introduction of curtains, painted or wall-paper patterns, and artwork at a level easily viewed from a wheelchair or a toddler's perspective further reduces the clinical aura of the treatment room setting.

Patient Rooms and the Pediatric Unit

Even as the child and family's first visual impression of the hospital itself is important, so too is the initial view of the unit where the child will stay. Does the child see a long, cluttered hallway, partially obscured by the glare of a distant window? Such a view reinforces a child's feelings of helplessness and insignificance in the face of a threatening new experience. How much more comforting it would be for the child to initially view an attractive play area or the pleasant vista of an outdoor greenspace. Explore ways of modifying the hallway decor to eliminate overwhelming expanses, conveying instead a feeling of warmth and acceptance to the family. For example, the length of a hallway may be more visually interesting if divided into sections painted different colors. Through the use of lighting, portions of the hallway, perhaps containing artwork at an appropriate level or manipulative activities attached to the wall, can be highlighted. Annoying glare from windows can be minimized through the use of tinted glass, blinds, and curtains.

Patient rooms should also be decorated in an attractive manner, with colorful walls, curtains, and carpeting. In addition to making the patient's room seem more home-like, carpeting further provides a warm, comfortable floor for the play of children. Ample wall-space should be provided in rooms for children to display their artistic creations, "get-well" cards, and posters. Walls to the hallway should be glazed to allow children to observe outside activity, an element particularly important when children are on bedrest or in isolation. To assure the privacy of patients, however, curtains should be provided around each patient's bed.

Since hospitalization is a largely passive experience for children, the ability to assert active control in the environment of their bedroom is all the more precious. The frequency with which some children use the nurse call button or change the channel on the television by remote control attests to this fact. When assessing the environment of a patient's room, observe the ways in which the setting promotes the child's activity and independence and formulate other means of enhancement. Does the child have access to storage space? Can the sink be operated from a wheel chair? Can children manipulate the room arrangement, moving chairs and beds (with the help of staff!) to a more comfortable arrangement? Are children free to place drawings and decorations throughout the room, or are they restricted to a small area or bulletin board? Any degree of control or decision-making power which can be vested in the child through the environment will help make hospitalization more palatable.

Upon completion of the environmental evaluation, the child life worker should discuss the findings with members of the department involved. Minor changes may be quickly and gratefully adopted by a staff too busy to have completed such an investigation themselves. At times the precise recommendation of the evaluator may prove unworkable, but the dialogue with staff members can lead to an acceptable alternative. Where child life workers believe the changes to be crucial, but more difficult to institute, they should present a proposal detailing implementation. A description of the problem, the impact of the proposed alteration, estimated cost, and sources of funding should be included in this document (see Chapter 10).

MONITORING OTHER ENVIRONMENTAL ELEMENTS

All too often, hospital personnel unknowingly create situations which are potentially harmful to children and their parents, when their intention is quite the opposite. A staff member will arrange for a costumed creature to visit the children as entertainment, but the resulting visit scares a group of toddlers at play. Or a nurse, intending to calm a mother's fears by providing an explicit explanation of her child's condition, uses overly graphic descriptions, alarming the child who overhears. In these, as with other elements of the environment, the child life worker should monitor the actions to insure that the best interests of the child are served.

Visiting Groups and Entertainment

The puppet troupe arrived with Dr. Clausson's highest recommendation. He had seen a portion of their Halloween performance at another hospital, and, impressed by what he termed "an utterly delightful show," made hasty arrangements for their appearance at Children's. By performance time the playroom was jammed with wheelchairs, IV poles, a gurney, and two traction beds, as children craned their necks or sat on parents' laps to slightly improve their view. The "utterly delightful show" that the children were to view contained, among other characters, a sea captain with one eye, a pirate whose severed hand had been replaced with a hook, and a rather gruesome looking ghost. Fortunately, more children appeared to leave the playroom due to boredom with the presentation than because of anxieties aroused through viewing the frightening, mutilated figures. One can only wonder what dreams the children had that night!

Special events such as plays, concerts, parties, and celebrity visits are exciting for hospitalized children, often representing the highlight of their hospital stay. Children who know that Cub Scouts are preparing a Valentine party or that a local sports hero will visit them have something to anticipate. These times are welcomed as a change from the routines of hospital life, and can benefit the children by offering them a chance to socialize much as they might outside of the hospital.

Problems can arise, however, when the nature of the entertainment is not fully understood by the hospital staff, or when the staff member arranging the event is not fully cognizant of the emotional needs and concerns of hospitalized children. As was the case in the puppet show described above, the entertainment may contain themes or characters that may unnecessarily frighten young patients. Children, for example, who are anticipating surgery and who may already harbor fears about the mutilation of their bodies have no need to view characters whose body parts are inexplicably absent. Plays treating themes which are likely to concern hospitalized children such as death or unresolved separation are inappropriate for hospital audiences, unless conducted with professional help as a means of helping selected groups of children deal with their feelings on the subject.

Costumes worn by visitors or their manner of approaching the children may easily upset the emotionally vulnerable patients. Even such benign characters as kings, queens, and fairy princesses may be threatening and incomprehensible to infants and toddlers. Others visitors such as clowns or "larger-than-life" cartoon characters may frighten even older patients by the antics so often considered essential to their roles. Before people such as these are permitted to tour the hospital or visit with patients, they should be informed of acceptable means of interacting with children, and they should be accompanied by a staff member who can direct them toward older children.

Much of the emotional peril to which children are exposed through the presence of unwittingly frightening entertainment can be eliminated if the duty to screen visitors is vested in the role of the child life worker. This policy should be known throughout the hospital, so that anyone who has knowledge of a possible presentation for children will refer this information to the child life staff. It is particularly important that the child life department gain the cooperation of the hospital's public relations director in this matter, since it is through that individual that many offers will be received.

When considering the merits of accepting the services of a particular individual or group, the child life staff should clarify a number of basic issues. Among these areas of concern are the following:

Type of Entertainment

When determining the nature of the entertainment, seek clarification of the type of activity involved and the age group to which it will likely appeal. A musical concert of contemporary tunes that might please a group of older children may prove boring to preschoolers, who would prefer hand-clapping to nursery rhymes. By knowing the specific type of entertainment to be presented, the child life staff can avoid scheduling an event for an entirely unsuitable audience.

At times, the type of entertainment suggested will cause the child life worker to probe more deeply into the content to assure that it is not objectionable from the child's perspective. For example, if a play is to be performed, what are the basic themes and characters? If a magic show, are any illusions excessively scary? In all cases, the child life worker should suggest that visiting groups plan to involve the patients actively in some way — singalongs, for example, rather than just providing passive entertainment.

Costumes

The wearing of costumes as part of a play or in conjunction with the visitation of children may be appealing and educational, as, for example, when the attire of other cultures or eras is modelled. However, before costumed individuals visit children, the types of costumes should be disclosed. Scary costumes, such as ghosts, skeletons, vampires or ferocious animals, should not be allowed. Questionable characters, such as clowns or other creatures whose actual faces are not readily visible, are likely to scare young patients. If allowed in the hospital at all, they should be confined to areas containing only older children, and they should be reminded to approach patients with gentleness.

Group Size

Excessive numbers of visitors may prove unworkable in a limited performance area, or, if visiting the children in their rooms, may dangerously overcrowd the hallways. A safe, acceptable number of visitors should be established. When arranging for entertainment, see that this limit is not exceeded.

Interaction with Patients

In addition to stressing the importance of visitors approaching patients in a nonthreatening manner, child life workers should also provide other guidelines for interaction with patients. The curious visitors may inquire of personnel or parents about the condition of patients, insensitive to the fact that the child is present to hear. (One of the authors remembers with pain standing with a member of the local professional football team, who was judging the annual Halloween costume contest at a children's hospital. As each patient paraded past, the visitor would turn and ask in a booming voice, "What's wrong with that kid? Why is he here?")

The obligatory phrase, "I hope you get well soon!" may be confusing to children who already consider themselves well. More troublesome is the comment from regular visitors, "I'll see you next week," when directed toward children who had been promised discharge at an earlier date. Visitors should be informed that concern for the patients is acceptable, but that it should not be expressed in a condescending manner, nor should it lead to a discussion of the patient's condition. Care should be taken by all visitors to avoid making promises to children that are not within their power to keep—for example, "I know that you'll be home very soon!"

Food Restrictions

Visiting groups and individuals should be reminded that many patients may be on restricted diets, and therefore they should not plan to distribute food indiscriminately. If the group is preparing a party for the children or plans refreshments with a performance, the child life staff must know about this in advance to suggest widely acceptable treats and to review the restrictions of patients.

Religious Content

The number of groups and individuals wishing to visit patients increases dramatically prior to holidays such as Christmas and Easter. Obviously, not all patients celebrate these holidays, and therefore the child life department should monitor proposed programming for religious content. The emphasis in such entertainment should be on multicultural celebrations, or spring or winter festivals, in which all patients may comfortably participate.

When members of a particular religious sect volunteer to perform some type of entertainment for the children, their assistance should be encouraged. The child life staff must, however, make it clear that the program should be for the benefit of all children, and should not promote a particular religious viewpoint.

Photographs

Many of the people volunteering their time to visit and entertain the children will wish to take pictures of the event—often as part of an attempt to gain publicity for themselves in the news media. Even when the pictures are for the personal use of the individual, the visitor must ask the child's or family's permission before they are taken. Most hospitals require that written permission be obtained also, particularly if the pictures have been taken for possible publication.

Other Considerations

The child life staff may find it necessary to formulate guidelines in other areas such as the length of stay of visitors or restriction of commercial promotion. These and all other policies should be communicated to the visitors prior to the scheduled entertainment.

An initial assessment of the suitability of the proposed entertainment should be made by a member of the child life staff through a conversation with a representative of the visiting group. At this time the policy considerations discussed above can be explained, and the child life worker can apprise the group of the conditions they are likely to encounter at the hospital, such as performance area, facilities, and the number of children generally participating in events of this type.

To insure that all visiting groups are aware of information discussed in the initial conversation, the child life department should send each group a copy of the departmental policies concerning such events. This information can be attached to a letter confirming the date and time of the group's arrival and performance, noting any special equipment requested by the group, and acknowledging the group's generosity in volunteering its time for the benefit of the children. By following a procedure of this sort, the child life department can increase the satisfaction of the performers and, more importantly, insure a beneficial experience for the hospitalized children.

Coordination of Patient Care

Another problem frequently noted by child life professionals is the failure to coordinate adequately the services of various departments. Unless an effort is made to schedule the access to patients by various professionals, a child can be easily overwhelmed by a succession of examinations by pediatricians, specialists, residents, and medical students, punctuated by a selection of diagnostic tests. The child is allowed no time to relax between events, and the opportunity to recapture a sense of mastery through play is rarely available. Meaningful preparation is sacrificed because of the limited time between procedures.

Easy solutions do not exist for a problem of this magnitude. A complex system of scheduling, coordinating the movements of numerous busy individuals, may be necessary, but will certainly not be easily accomplished. To relax the pace of demands on children, an earlier admission may be essential, an unpopular recommendation in many quarters because of the accelerating cost of a hospital stay.

Although the problems may seem insurmountable, the child life worker who observes the hazards of this situation should not be dissuaded from seeking change. Certainly the task cannot be accomplished alone. An ideal forum for exploration of this problem is in the interdisciplinary meetings of the health care team (see Chapter 8). Here the ideas of the individuals involved in providing care to the children can be expressed and workable solutions explored.

Communication and the Child

Attempts to serve children and their parents through the provision of accurate information are, indeed, laudable. At times, however, the intention may be good, but the means of execution is misguided. Among the more common problems of this sort are the following:

Talking in the Presence of Children

Professionals frequently proceed with explanations to parents concerning a child's condition or a forthcoming procedure, insensitive to the child's presence. This in itself is demeaning to children, conveying to them that they are unworthy of receiving a personal explanation. This condition can be even more hazardous when the speaker, assuming that the child is either not attending to the explanation or is incapable of understanding it, proceeds with a discussion of sensitive information. Young children, although their skills of verbal expression may be limited, are capable of understanding a great deal. Through a combination of those words comprehended and the concerned looks of the speaker and parents, the child can easily gain enough to provoke anxieties and spur fantasies.

Using Overly Graphic Language

Even when the communications of professionals are appropriately directed toward parent or child, problems may arise from the speaker's choice of words. Certain words, though accurate in conveying meaning, are charged with excessive emotional content and should therefore be avoided. When offering explanations to children, Petrillo and Sanger (1980) suggest that the staff "use neutral words like opening, draining and oozing instead of cut and bleed (p. 235)." Likewise, anesthesia should not be described as making children be "put to sleep" since this phrasing may remind the child of the fate of a family pet.

At times staff members try to make an explanation more comprehensible to children by referring to objects or describing procedures in terms of animate objects, or, conversely, describing human organs in inanimate terms. Thus a catheterization might be referred to as "a snake going through your body," or the urinary tract as "plumbing." The literal-minded preschooler, so prone to belief in fantastic explanations always, can only be further confused or frightened by these misguided word choices.

Offering Choices Where None Exist

"Do you want to take your medicine now?" "Is it all right if I give you your shot now?" "Would you like to come to the treatment room with me?" Questions such as these are frequently heard throughout the hospital, often followed by the very honest response from a child: "No!" It is unfair to offer what may seem to children like choices when, in reality, none exist. Staff members must turn these questions into statements, coupling them with *realistic* choices whenever possible. For example, "It's time for your medicine. Would you like it with water or juice?" or "It's time for your shot; which arm should I use?" By proceeding in this manner, the staff allows the child to retain a degree of mastery, and avoids the loss of trust which often results from having requested responses ignored.

Many of the communication problems described above arise as a result of ignorance. Staff members may not be aware of the power of their language or of the ability of young children to comprehend verbal or nonverbal communication. Phrases such as "Can I give you your shot now?" are more likely repeated out of mindless habit, rather than in a conscious attempt to deceive children. If staff members are made aware of the effect of their communications on the children, offered in the spirit of constructive criticism, they may be more than willing to alter their patterns for the benefit of patients. When communication problems are particularly pervasive among personnel, or it is difficult to directly change the patterns of certain staff members, workshops on the improvement of the communication process may be organized.

Rounds

A common occurrence on hospital wards is the daily session of medical rounds. A group of physicians tour the hospital unit, examining patients and noting their progress. Generally, there is a teaching component to the rounds, as residents are given an opportunity to examine and discuss the condition of patients displaying a variety of diagnoses. While a valuable experience from the perspective of medical education, rounds are a potential nightmare for the unsuspecting child. Numerous white-coated figures surround the child's bed, talking in hushed serious tones. The physicians take turns thrusting hands and instruments toward the child performing their individual examinations. Unless managed properly, medical rounds can be an overwhelming and threatening experience which unnecessarily subjects children to potential harm through misinterpretation of information overheard.

Child life workers who find the rounds procedure damaging to children in their individual settings may attempt to intervene by helping the child prepare for the experience and by suggesting alterations in the format for rounds. Petrillo and Sanger (1980) suggest that all children hospitalized for the first time be briefed on the meaning of rounds. Children can be told what to expect during the procedure and can be told that the number of doctors present does not indicate the severity of the child's condition or that treatment has gone wrong.

In addition, physicians should be made aware of the impact of entering a child's room en masse, treating the child impersonally, and talking in such a manner that children can easily overhear. This may be graphically presented to physicians through the words of children, e.g. through the tape-recorded comments or written stories, and their drawings of the experience. A few simple, yet effective guidelines may be offered to decrease the difficulty of rounds for children. For example, major discussion of the child's condition should not occur in the room or in the doorway. The number of participants should be limited, and the child should be introduced to each. Petrillo and Sanger (1980) urge professionals participating in rounds to interact with the children in a personal manner, apologizing for the interruption and commenting on the child's interests.

Lindheim et al. (1972) suggest more fundamental changes in the process of conducting rounds, such as the installation of closed circuit television cameras in patient rooms and the utilization of a demonstration treatment room with one-way mirrors for observers to look through. By using these mechanisms, children could be examined by a single individual or small group of familiar people, with others observing elsewhere. Through the use of videotape cameras, examinations could be recorded for use at other times. A small meeting room near each pediatric unit for discussion following the examination would reduce the likelihood of a child overhearing provocative information.

In many settings medical and nursing rounds are well entrenched, nearly sacred traditions, which may prove difficult to change, but their potential for harming children is so great that the offending practices should not be allowed to proceed unaltered.

Summary

Children and their families enter the hospital in an emotionally vulnerable state. Every contact families have with the hospital, either through interaction with hospital personnel or encounters with elements of the hospital environment have the capacity to increase or diminish the concerns of the individual. Through a systematic evaluation of the hospital environment, a continual monitoring of those elements of greatest concern, and frequent presentation to other staff members of the viewpoint of children and their families, the child life workers help assure the positive, caring nature of those contacts.

CHAPTER 8

RELATIONS WITH OTHER PROFESSIONALS

WORKING IN THE HOSPITAL CONTEXT

The modern hospital is a labyrinthine institution, as intricate in its organizational structure as in its architectural design. Hundreds of highly skilled professionals, each expert in such diverse fields as marketing research, radiation therapy, and community resources, combine efforts in the delivery of quality health care to patients. The intense specialization in today's health care facilities is a phenomenon of relatively recent origin. When the Hospital for Sick Children in Great Ormand Street (England's first children's hospital) was established in London in 1852, its founder, Dr. Charles West, not only served as physician-in-chief but also furnished the building, wrote the hospital's catalogue, and organized the accounting system (Love, Henderson, & Stewart, 1972).

While specialization of services allows individual professionals to master increasingly complex subject matter and to apply that knowledge in support of the patient's health, it also entails problems that may inhibit optimum patient care. The division of medical and nonmedical functions into ever-smaller units results in a corresponding proliferation of hospital personnel. A patient admitted for minor surgery may encounter several individuals from the admitting department and business office; laboratory, X-ray, and EKG technicians; an array of nurses working three shifts; and physicians, including residents, surgeons, anesthesiologists, and other specialists. Incidental contacts with personnel from housekeeping, maintenance, dietary, and volunteer services are inevitable. While forced interaction with so many individuals may be disconcerting to an adult patient, it is potentially devastating for the young child whose entire world had previously consisted of a handful of close people.

Inherent in the decentralization of patient care are problems of communication. With the involvement of an increased number of professionals in the care of a given patient comes the potential of transmitting contradictory information. Each views the treatment of the patient from a slightly different perspective and may, therefore, possess different opinions on the proper course to be pursued. Accurate exchange of information through patient charts and regularly scheduled team meetings permits resolution of major conflicts in the approach to patient care. By establishing a unified course of action, the health care team minimizes the patient's anxiety and inevitable loss of trust engendered by the dissemination of conflicting views from different individuals.

The complexity of modern hospitals also has implications for the institution of necessary changes. As with any large organization, the alteration of programs or services of a hospital frequently involves slow and laborious activity as a proposal moves from one committee to another gathering necessary approval. Without an understanding of hospital organization or possession of the interpersonal skills essential to generate support, the effecting of change becomes an impossible task.

If child life workers are to serve as effective advocates for children and their families, implementing change as needed, they must possess a sophisticated knowledge of hospital organization and cultivate functional relationships with professionals in other disciplines. Continual communication with others involved in the care of children, via notations in patients' charts and participation in team meetings, informs other professionals of the emotional needs of individual children and defines the broader goals of child life programming.

Hospital organization and the roles of various professionals within the organization will be examined in the present chapter. Means of enhancing communications between the child life department and other disciplines, as well as strategies for coping with potential resistance to child life programming from those areas, will also be explored.

UNDERSTANDING HOSPITAL STRUCTURE AND PERSONNEL

Hospital Organization

The organizational structure of each hospital and the departments it comprises will, of course, vary with the nature of the hospital and its philosophy of management. A long-term care facility for children may, for example, place a greater emphasis on rehabilitative services than a general hospital and may entirely eliminate a surgical unit. Organizationally, some hospitals adopt a strictly heirarchical "chain of command" with certain departments subordinate to others. In other facilities a number of departments are placed on an equal organizational level, each having direct access to a superior. The following illustration depicts a combination of these two approaches, with those departments under the Assistant Administrator for Operations forming a hierarchical pyramid, while those under the Assistant Administrator for Patient Care displaying a "flatter" configuration. The departments considered in this chapter (those shown in the following illustration) are typical of those found in most facilities serving children.

Board of Trustees

Formation of hospital policy lies with the board of trustees or board of directors, a group of individuals selected from the community, who

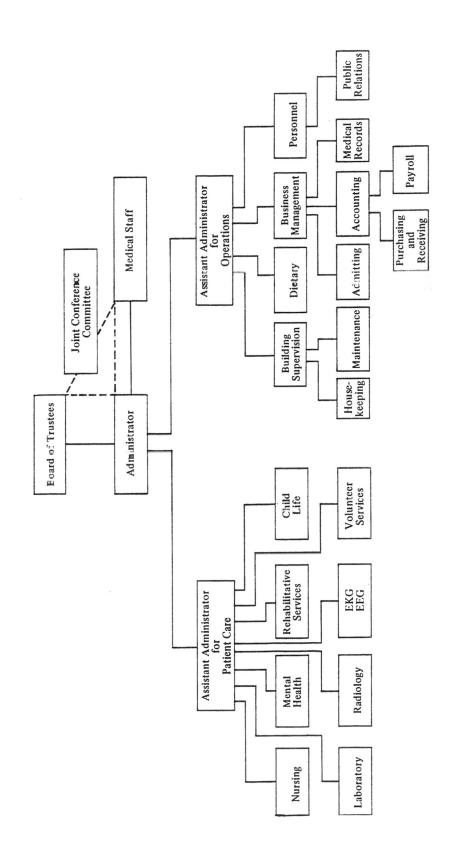

volunteer their time to supervise the broad aspects of hospital operations. This group is ultimately responsible for the financial stability and professional quality of the institution. Through appointment of an administrator, the medical staff, and various committees, its policies are enacted. An executive committee, composed of officers of the board, is frequently empowered to act in place of the board during the period between board meetings.

Communication between the board, the administrator, and the medical staff is often maintained through a "joint conference committee," generally comprised of equal numbers of board members and physicians, plus the administrator. In this body recommendations for policy changes, new appointments to the staff, and other issues are discussed before presentation to the entire board.

Medical Staff

Physicians associated with a given hospital constitute the medical staff. This group is further subdivided into smaller units according to the nature of the physician's association with the hospital. The *honorary medical staff* consists of distinguished professionals who hold appointment elsewhere or who formerly practiced in the hospital but have now retired. This group has no active role in the hospital. The *consulting medical staff* includes physicians who are recognized specialists in their fields. These individuals are available for consultation upon request from the hospital's active medical staff. Physicians not regularly members of the hospital staff, but wishing to hospitalize their private patients in the facility, compose the *courtesy staff*. Formulation of major medical policy is the responsibility of the *active medical staff*, through elected officers and established committees. Members of the active medical staff inform and influence governing board decisions through participation on the joint conference committee.

In addition to these physicians, many hospitals have a *resident medical staff*, consisting of physicians who treat patients as part of their graduate medical education. These doctors-in-training make up what is sometimes referred to as the *house staff* or *house officers*. Private physicians are then called the *attending staff* or *attendings*.

Administration

The individual appointed by the Board of Trustees to serve as executive officer implementing its policies is the *hospital administrator*. The administrator is charged with coordinating the functions and activities of the hospital's various departments, making management decisions concerning the allocation and addition of personnel and equipment, and monitoring the hospital's financial status. A major responsibility of the administrator is insuring the hospital's compliance with regulations promulgated by government agencies concerning the delivery of health care.

The hospital administrator maintains an active community involvement, promoting the hospital, interpreting its programs and mission, and seeking sources of funds. Supervision of portions of the hospital's operation may be delegated to one or more assistant administrators.

Hospital Operations

A number of the hospital's departments serve a supportive role in the facility's operation, providing for its day-to-day functioning and making it possible to care for patients, while not being directly involved in that care. Contacts between members of these departments (shown in the diagram as reporting to the Assistant Administrator for Operations) and patients is generally of an informal nature, if it occurs at all. Noteworthy exceptions are members of the admitting department, who are among the first to greet children upon arrival at the hospital, and dieticians or nutritionists who frequently consult with children and parents.

Business Manager

The hospital, ultimately, is a business, albeit a nonprofit business. Its successful operation will, to a large extent, depend upon the application of sound business principles. For this reason, the business manager (who may also be called director of finances, controller, or business service director, among other titles) serves an important role in hospital operations. The individual occupying this position advises the Administrator and the Board of Trustees on financial matters, establishes accounting procedures for the hospital, and frequently serves as administrator for other departments such as purchasing, accounting, and admitting.

Admitting Department

In a strictly functional role, personnel employed in the admitting department gather information on patients and their families to facilitate other aspects of the patient's care. Rooms are often assigned through this department, old patient records obtained, and the availability of necessary facilities such as operating rooms verified. The admitting department also compiles a daily census report.

The admitting department's impact on patient care, however, goes far beyond the performance of these essential duties. As perhaps the first member of the hospital staff with whom parents and children have contact upon arrival, admitting personnel are in a position to set the tone for the family's hospital stay. By directing attention to the child and asking questions of parents in a sensitive, compassionate manner, the admitting clerk conveys a positive image of the hospital from the earliest moments of encounter. The interviewing skills of an admitting clerk must be particularly keen when dealing with overly anxious parents or when admitting a child under emergency conditions. Failure to handle these delicate situations properly may provoke parental hostility toward the hospital, impeding the formation of a trusting relationship with other members of the hospital staff.

Medical Records

Careful records are compiled on every patient who enters the hospital. The medical records administrator develops a system for storing this massive amount of information and retrieving it when patients are readmitted. The staff working under the direction of the administrator transcribes physicians' notes concerning patient care, codes the information recorded in patients' charts according to various classifications such as diagnoses or method of treatment, and compiles statistics to evaluate patient care and services, based on that information. All information found in patients' permanent records must be reviewed by medical records personnel to insure accuracy and completeness.

Other Business Offices

The hospital *accounting department* performs the bookkeeping functions for the institution, maintaining records on daily receipts, accounts receivable, the employee payroll, and other hospital expenses. Closely associated with the accounting department is the *payroll department*, which processes employee time sheets, calculates taxes and other deductions from earnings, and issues paychecks, maintaining thorough and accurate records of all transactions.

All supplies necessary for the operation of the complex hospital institution are obtained by the *purchasing department* and *receiving department*. Requests for materials are received by the purchasing department, which places orders with companies based on market research to determine the most advantageous price. After the items purchased are received by the hospital, they must be stored, periodically inventoried, and distributed to the requesting department as needed.

Personnel

The personnel officer of a hospital is charged with attracting the best possible talent to the institution and matching those individuals with the appropriate position. This frequently involves initial interviewing and screening of applicants for a given job, the most qualified of whom are referred to the appropriate department head for final selection. In addition to this function, the personnel staff analyze existing positions within the institution, retaining an accurate job description of each. Employee compensation is based on the skills and responsibilities reflected by these descriptions.

The personnel department is responsible for the employee's orientation to the hospital and establishes a set of guidelines or policies concerning the hiring, advancement, and termination of personnel. These guidelines further delineate relationships among personnel and benefit afforded employees by the hospital.

Public Relations

It is the function of the public relations director to convey a positive image of the hospital and its services to the community. This may be accomplished through the use of television, radio, newspaper and magazine stories depicting unique services and events, or highlighting particular employees. The public relations department is also responsible for the production of information and pamphlets distributed to patients and personnel describing various aspects of the hospital's function.

As discussed in the previous chapter, it is essential for the child life staff to maintain a close working relationship with public relations personnel. The pediatric unit, and child life activities in particular, provide many opportunities for media coverage that would increase the visibility of the hospital and enhance its image within the community. A story presented in a sensitive manner may prove beneficial in educating the public about the goals of child life programming and the needs of hospitalized children. The child life staff must, however, guard against frequent or inappropriate intrusions into the lives of patients. The welfare of patients must always remain paramount.

Child life personnel also work with the public relations staff in the development of educational materials for children and their parents, insuring that the material presented is accurate and is presented in a clear and supportive manner.

Dietary Department

The task of planning menus for patients, managing food supplies, and preparing and serving meals is the responsibility of the dietary department. A large portion of the functioning of this department is never viewed by the children, who only see the final product of dietary's efforts arrive at mealtime. As previously suggested, the food preparation facilities provide an excellent focus for a patient field trip arranged by the child life staff. Members of the child life department may further use their contacts with the dietary staff to suggest changes in children's menus or to make arrangements for special cooking projects.

A dietician or nutritionist frequently operates as a member of the primary patient health care team, advising patients on changes in diets necessitated by illness such as diabetes, and teaching sound nutritional practices.

Maintenance Department

The tremendous task of maintaining the hospital's physical plant, repairing broken machinery, and assuring that the vital systems transmitting electricity, heat, water, and oxygen supplies to all areas of the building rests with the maintenance staff. Staff members generally include plumbers, electricians, painters, and engineers.

Child life contact with personnel from the maintenance staff will prove valuable in many ways. The shop, with its array of tools and machinery, presents another prime location for an in-hospital field trip. Furthermore, the maintenance work area is an excellent source of scrap wood, snips of wire, discarded tile and dozens of other materials to fuel the art projects of young patients. One girl, for example, completed an intricate doll house, furnished with tiny furniture and wall-to-wall carpeting, with materials located by maintenance personnel and no small amount of labor donated by the shop staff from lunch hours and breaks.

Environmental Services

The interior of the hospital must not only be kept hazard-free and presentable, it must also be thoroughly cleaned following precise guidelines to prevent the spread of infection. The environmental services department, or housekeeping staff, has the responsibility for completing this task. The director of this department in consultation with other staff members establishes cleaning procedures designed to minimize the possibility of cross-contamination, and trains housekeeping personnel in their use. In addition, the director of environmental services frequently determines the types of furnishings permissible in the hospital setting; basing that decision on the item's function, its safety, and ability to be cleaned. The child life worker selecting playroom furnishings or other materials should consult with this individual to insure that articles desired are acceptable and to avoid the substitution of other items which, although permissible from an infection control perspective, fail to meet the needs of the children. The differences in an alternate selection of an art table may appear negligible to the environmental services director, but if the slight differences impede access by children in wheelchairs, they are critical.

Patient Care

Another category of hospital departments includes those services that are more directly involved in the care of the patient, providing medical or emotional support to children and their families. Child life contact with these departments is generally more frequent, and often more formal in nature, than the interaction with departments previously discussed. Individuals from many of the patient care departments will, along with the child life staff, form the health care team responsible for the primary care of the patient.

Nursing Service

The major portion of the direct patient care in a hospital is provided by nursing service. Members of the nursing staff assist in the formulation of a treatment plan and carry out procedures prescribed by the physician. They observe the patients, noting symptoms and reactions to treatments and assessing patient progress, carefully recording their observations in the patient's chart. Throughout the course of their interactions with patients and their families, nurses provide instructions about procedures and the proper use of medications and offer emotional support to those in their care.

The nursing service, commonly the largest department in the hospital, is administered by a registered nurse, the *director of nursing*, who is charged with general planning, supervision, and assessment of the entire nursing staff. The director of nursing plays an important role in the formulation and implementation of nursing policies and procedures. The magnitude of the supervisory task demanded of this position may require the presence of one or more *assistant directors of nursing.*

Nursing supervisors are responsible for the direct supervision of nursing activities in a portion of the hospital consisting of several individual units, each having its own *head nurse*. Within an individual hospital unit, it is the head nurse who is responsible for the coordination of patient care, assigning nurses to patients, reviewing the written orders of physicians, and supervising the reporting of observations by the nursing staff. In the absence of the head nurse, a *charge nurse* assumes responsibility for coordination of the nursing staff within a unit.

In addition to the certified nursing staff (Registered Nurses and Licensed Practical Nurses [LPN's], who must practice under the supervision of a physician or RN), the nursing service employs nurses aides, orderlies, and/or clerks, who perform nonprofessional aspects of nursing care, thereby allowing the nurses to apply their skills in a more efficient and appropriate fashion.

Child life contact with the nursing staff should be close and continual, if patients are to receive optimal care. Instances of a child's resistance to medication, excessive fear of injections, or anxious behavior following the departure of a parent are observed countless times daily by members of the nursing staff. In these and other situations the child life worker should be notified so that appropriate interventions may be made. Conversely, insights acquired during sessions with the child life staff must be transmitted to the nursing staff if the observations are to benefit the child. Mechanisms for enhancing verbal and written communication will be discussed more fully later in this chapter.

Mental Health Professions

Closely allied with the goals of the child life department are those of the mental health professions. The health of a patient is not solely dependent on the resolution of a medical condition. Frequently a parent's condition is either partially the product of, or is aggravated by, conditions in the individual's environment. A baby eats chips of the faded paint peeling from the walls of a family's deteriorating apartment and contacts lead poisoning. Or a mother, deterred by the cost of medical care, neglects to seek treatment for a child's sore until a severe infection develops. These conditions may be treated medically, but unless the families of these children receive help in dealing with broader socioeconomic problems, similar situations are likely to occur. The *social service department*, whose members are informed about community resources and understand the dynamics of family relationships, can intervene in such cases, making referrals to appropriate agencies and counseling with individuals and families.

The departments of *psychiatry* and *psychology* function in a similar manner, attempting to control or eliminate psychological factors contributing to the disease process and ameliorating the emotional stress resulting from a patient's condition. Most hospitals also provide a *pastoral care department*. Hospital chaplains are available to provide spiritual and emotional support and counseling to hospitalized children and their families.

Since the role of the child life worker is so inextricably linked with the emotional life of children and their families, communication with these professions is crucial. Because of the freedom inherent in the play situation, the child life staff will frequently observe children expressing vital concerns or will watch the interaction of children with their parents. Information gained in this manner can, if relayed to the appropriate professional, prove valuable in detecting and eliminating problems which present barriers to children.

Rehabilitative Services

Many children who enter the hospital will, because of the nature of these conditions, come in contact with one of several specialized therapists. The skills of these individuals help children regain full strength and capacities diminished by the illness.

Physical therapists work with children who have suffered muscular, skeletal, or nerve damage as a result of disease or injury. Through a series of diagnostic tests, the physical therapist assesses the strength, coordination, and development of the individual and, in consultation with the physician, develops a treatment plan. The patient's treatment may consist of an exercise program and application of heat, cold, light, water, or electrical stimuli to the weakened area. Patients permanently impaired receive practice and instruction in techniques designed to provide them with maximum self-sufficiency.

Frequently working in tandem with physical therapists are *occupational therapists*. Motion and abilities restored through the physical therapy process are translated into workable skills through occupational therapy. These professionals evaluate the skills of patients and develop a treatment plan accordingly. Through the use of activities and with the assistance of specially designed adaptive devices, the occupational therapists help the individual become as self-sufficient as possible within limitations presented by the patient's condition.

The role of the *respiratory therapist*, or inhalation therapist, is not confined to the rehabilitative mode, although these professionals do provide instructions and demonstrate techniques designed to aid victims of chronic respiratory problems. Respiratory therapists may also intervene in emergency situations, such as poisonings or head injuries, resulting in acute respiratory distress. Failure to restore an adequate supply of oxygen to the patient within a few minutes could result in death or permanent brain damage.

Surgical patients whose breathing may be hampered due to the nature of the operation may also receive assistance from the respiratory therapist. Working with the patient's physician, the respiratory therapist may employ equipment such as respirators or positive-pressure breathing machines to provide temporary breathing assistance.

Laboratory Personnel

The accurate detection and diagnosis of a patient's condition is an essential prerequisite to effective treatment. The function of the hospital laboratory is to assist in this investigative process through the analysis of human tissue, blood, urine, and other body fluids. Working under the general supervision of a *pathologist* (a physician who diagnoses the causes of disease), *medical technologists* and *medical technicians* perform numerous tests to identify the nature of a patient's medical condition and to direct the proper course of treatment.

The most visible representatives of the hospital's laboratory are those individuals who have the thankless duty of drawing blood samples from frequently unwilling young patients. The unsuccessful or difficult blood drawing represents a singularly traumatic experience for the hospitalized child. It is painful and frightening, and is often accompanied by the increasing frustration and anger of flustered staff members. A child's fantasy that the procedure is a grisly form of punishment is reinforced by the admonition from laboratory personnel that, "If you don't hold still,

I'll have to do it again!" While this may, in fact, be the case, the frightened child hearing these words may translate them as "If you don't submit, I'll have to hurt you again to teach you a lesson!"

The laboratory worker participating in this scene is no more pleased with the struggle than the terrified child. Communication between the child life worker and laboratory personnel can reduce much of this strife. Many common childhood fantasies surround blood tests, among them are beliefs that all blood will be removed or that a permanent hole will be left in the patient's arm. Needle play and preparation for the tests may reveal and correct such misconceptions. The child life worker making such observations during the course of medical play should relate these findings to laboratory personnel, who can watch for their reemergence and offer reassurance as needed. The child life worker and laboratory personnel should further discuss strategies for approaching children and assisting them with the procedure. The presence of a child's parents and the ability to make even such limited choices as designating the finger or arm from which blood will be drawn restore a feeling of security and control to the child.

Radiology Department

A large percentage of patients entering the hospital have contact with the department of radiology, principally to have X-ray pictures, or *radiographs*, taken for diagnostic or screening purposes. Treatment of a fractured bone, the location of a tumor, or determination of the severity of a patient's pneumonia are all made possible through the examination of radiographs. Hospitals, however, use radiation for purposes beyond the ordinary X-rays. In *nuclear medicine*, radioactive materials are applied to the patient, frequently through intravenous injection, for diagnostic purposes. The rays emitted are recorded on sophisticated machinery that allows radiologists (physicians who specialize in the use of radiation) to better evaluate the functioning of internal organs. In *radiation therapy*, various forms of radiation are used in the treatment of diseases, most commonly cancer.

Although radiologists are responsible for reading X-rays, making diagnoses, and recommending treatment, it is the X-ray technologists and technicians with whom patients have most contact. The majority of X-ray procedures commonly performed in the hospital are not invasive; that is, they do not require the patient to ingest anything or to receive an injection. The procedures, nevertheless, may be extremely frightening to the child who does not understand what is happening or is treated in an insensitive manner. As is the case with laboratory personnel, the child life worker can consult with the X-ray department staff, transmitting information revealed during play sessions and discussing appropriate means of helping children cope with radiologic procedures.

EKG and EEG

The hospitalized patient's condition may require the use of other specialized tests to obtain an accurate diagnosis. The *electrocardiograph* (EKG) records electric impulses emitted by the heart as it contracts. The physician may examine the tracings, or electrocardiogram, to assess the condition of the heart and to detect irregularities in its function. To conduct this procedure, an EKG technician straps electrodes to the patient's chest, arms, and legs, manipulating the chest electrodes to record different readings of the heart's action.

The electrical activity of the brain may be recorded for diagnostic purposes by a machine called an *electroencephalograph*. The EEG test is primarily performed on patients suspected of having a neurological disorder such as a stroke, brain tumor, or seizures. The technician conducting the test attaches electrodes to various parts of the patient's head, and adjusts the machine to obtain the type of recording desired.

While neither of these procedures is painful, both can be terrifying for children who are unfamiliar with the machinery and the threatening electrodes. It is essential that children who face these examinations be prepared for the experience, playing through the procedure with models of the equipment. Failure to inform children adequately of the nature and purpose of the procedure leaves them vulnerable to horrible fantasies, often promoted by visions of science-fiction laboratories. In addition to overseeing the preparation, the child life worker should consult with EKG and EEG personnel concerning their interaction with children.

Volunteer Services

Individuals who donate their services perform a variety of important functions necessary to the operation of the hospital. Volunteers serve as receptionists, messengers, and companions for patients. They also assist the paid hospital staff by transporting patients, doing clerical work, or serving in more specialized functions, such as establishing a library for patients, leading hospital tours, or conducting playroom sessions. These individuals generally work under the supervision of a paid member of the hospital staff, the *director of volunteer services*, who is responsible for their recruitment and orientation.

Since the duties of many volunteers will lead to contact and interaction with children, and their prior experience with children may be limited, the child life staff should assist the director of volunteer services in preparing orientation and training sessions. Reactions of children to hospitalization should be stressed, and guidelines for appropriate dealings with patients and their families delineated.

The preceding pages briefly examined many of the major disciplines found in hospitals serving children. This catalog is by no means exhaustive (a fact which, in itself, testifies to the complexity of hospitals). The relations and communication between those departments working closely with children and the child life staff will be explored more fully in the following section.

COMMUNICATION WITH OTHER PROFESSIONALS

Communicating with Departments Having Brief Contact with Children

As indicated in the previous section, many individuals throughout the hospital have frequent, though brief, encounters with hospitalized children. Admitting personnel initially greet children and their families upon arrival at the hospital, perhaps not seeing them again until discharge. Laboratory workers perform dozens of blood tests on individual children daily, with each lasting no more than a few minutes. A similar situation prevails for EKG or X-ray technicians, who serve a large number of children during the day and have limited contact with each.

The brevity of these contacts handicaps health care workers who must seek the cooperation of children for the successful completion of a procedure. Personnel from the various departments that serve children under such circumstances have virtually no opportunity to know the children as individuals, gaining a sense of the unique concerns of each. Much needless anxiety to the child and the staff member as well can be avoided if all hospital personnel are aware of

(1) typical reactions of children of various ages to contact with strangers and the performance of medical procedures

(2) communication skills, for offering effective explanations of events to children of all ages and for initially contacting children in a nonthreatening manner

(3) the particular concerns of individual children.

Through the presentation of inservices to health care workers and the development of educational materials, the child life staff can provide information on the first two categories. Personnel from departments such as X-ray, EKG, or EEG are frequently surprised to learn that children often view their procedures as punishment. Yet once they have attained this awareness, they are better able to appreciate the discomfort of children in their presence, and can offer reassurance that the procedure is necessary to help rather than punish them.

A few simple words of advice on communication skills can be of tremendous help in facilitating the interaction between child and staff. Initially contacting children when parents are present, kneeling down to the level of a child when talking, and investing a few minutes in play with the child to establish rapport help prevent an immediate hostile reaction that makes the completion of a procedure difficult if not impossible.

The child life staff can also assist members of other disciplines who have limited contact with children by transmitting information about the personality of individual children or the nature of their particular concerns. If, for example, a child reveals a hatred of lying down while blood is drawn, preferring to sit upright instead, this information should be communicated to the laboratory staff.

The exact nature of the communication process may take several forms. Child life notations in the patient's chart or in the written nursing care plan (or "Kardex®") may be reviewed by others having contact with the child. Information which specifically applies to a given discipline should be communicated directly to the personnel involved, as well as being entered in the written records. Personnel in the X-ray department, for example, should be notified if the play of a child scheduled for an X-ray procedure includes the use of laser beams and "death rays." (Note: If, in a situation of this sort, the child appears overly anxious and in need of greater intervention than a reinforcement of preparation and reassurance of the benign nature of the procedure, the event should be postponed to allow for further exploration and allaying of the child's fears.)

Communication should not flow solely from the child life staff to other disciplines. Child life workers must consult with members of other departments to gain an understanding of procedures performed in each. Without this knowledge it is impossible to prepare children adequately for forthcoming experiences. Furthermore, the child life staff must rely on the personnel performing procedures for information concerning those children who experienced difficulty during the process. The child who found an EKG test upsetting (and who may be in need of more such examinations in the near future) requires child life intervention to work through anxieties aroused by the event. Play may reveal the fantasy producing the adverse reaction and allow the child to regain a sense of mastery over the frightening events, thereby helping the child cope with repetition of the procedure at a future time.

Communicating with the Primary Health Care Team

Those professionals participating in the direct, ongoing physical and emotional care of children and their families constitute the health care team. The number of people working with a given patient will, of course, vary with that child's physical condition, emotional strength, and social environment, but the health care team generally consists of physicians, nurses, social workers, psychologists, chaplain, and child life workers. Rehabilitative therapists, dieticians, or other specialists may also be involved in the team's activities. Through formal and informal communication, members of the health care team coordinate their activities, identify problems in the treatment of patients (assigning individual members to intervene according to the nature of their skills), and explore new ways of improving patient care.

During regularly scheduled team conferences, the care of children on a nursing unit is reviewed. Observations made by team members are shared, frequently revealing conditions about which no one individual was aware. For instance, a child's seemingly normal comment to a chaplain that "my mommy won't come back," and the child life worker's observation that the child's play revealed themes of abandonment take on new significance when coupled with a social worker's suspicion, based on a conversation with the mother, that the children are left at home by themselves for long periods of time. Rather than merely evidencing a concern common to many hospitalized children, this child's actions may indicate problems of a more serious nature at home. Once members of the health care team have identified a problem in this manner, efforts to manage the problem may be discussed and coordinated.

In addition to the regularly scheduled conferences, members may arrange special meetings to plan the care of children whose problems are particularly complex. For example, a patient hospitalized for an extended period of time who will require extensive care at home upon discharge may be the subject of an additional care conference. The child's time in the hospital must be structured to prevent excessive boredom, and the expression of his feelings concerning his condition should be encouraged. Educational experiences while hospitalized must be arranged, and specialized equipment necessary for use at home obtained. If the parents are of modest means and lack adequate insurance coverage, financial matters must be addressed. The child's parents may also require ongoing emotional support to help them cope with the stress of having a child with major medical problems. Having identified the major foreseeable problems, members of the health care team can then develop a comprehensive care plan to meet the physical and emotional needs of the child and family.

Due to the difficulties of coordinating the schedules of a number of professionals, the health care team meetings will likely be held no more often than once or twice weekly. Since only limited amounts of information can be transmitted during these meetings, and since they will not be able to deal with children who are admitted and discharged in the intervening period, other forms of inter-professional communication must be employed. The child life worker should record all important observations concerning the behavior of children in the patient's permanent record. Here it is available for other team members to read and comment upon.

Additionally, child life workers should schedule daily brief report sessions with the head nurse from their unit, to review the needs of children. Since the nursing staff spend more time with the children than any other discipline, their observations of patients' reactions to hospitalization and treatment are invaluable to the child life worker attempting to identify those children whose needs are most acute. Their intensive contact with children also means that they have greater opportunity to benefit from the observations of the child life staff. During the daily report sessions insights derived from the child life worker's play and interaction with children can be transmitted to the nursing staff.

The use of a child life report sheet, such as that shown in Table I, may prove valuable in organizing child life interventions and transferring information to the nursing staff during the report sessions. Under the "Problems" column, the child life worker can record special concerns for each child noted by the nursing staff. For example, the problem may be a child's incapacitating fear of injections. As a possible intervention, the child life worker might attempt to engage the child in needle play. Following the needle play, the child life worker can note the results in the "Outcome and Observations" column. Information recorded on the child life report sheet serves as the basis for notations placed in the child's chart or written nursing care plan.

The child life report sheet serves an additional purpose, particularly important for individuals establishing child life programming where none had previously existed. For nursing staff not familiar with child life programming, the report sheet is an educational tool demonstrating the range of child life interventions. Whenever a new problem is revealed by the nursing staff, the child life worker can suggest means of coping with the situation, thereby continually expanding nursing's understanding of the activities that child life workers utilize.

Communication through Written Records

Two primary mechanisms exist for communicating in written form with members of other disciplines: the patient's permanent record, or chart, and the nursing care plan, or "Kardex®." To use these instruments effectively, the child life worker must understand their structure and function.

The Chart

The precise format of the patient's record is determined by the individual hospital, but most charts contain the following major sections:

(1) *The admitting sheet* contains basic information such as the patient's name, age, address, parents' names, etc. Also included is the physician's tentative diagnosis at the time of admission.

(2) *The history section* includes the patient's medical history, describing the present illness, past medical data, as well as medical and social history of the patient's family. The results of a complete physical exami-

TABLE I

CHILD LIFE REPORT FORM

Child Life Worker:_____   Date:_____

Name Room	Age Diagnosis	Problems	Possible Interventions	Outcome and Observations
Tim Wescott 114 B	3 fx. rt femur	Immobility due to traction not tolerated well.	Put posters on ceiling Bring in toys with movable parts; fishbowl & fish Imaginative play Rig ball on string	Watched fish intently for 10 minutes; periodically watched them later Laughed when he played with the ball. Traction needed adjustment once during morning
Janie Calder 115 A	5 Appendectomy	(1) Isolation	(1) Medical play; assess understanding of isolation Assign volunteer to spend time w/patient Telephone contact w/other patients	(1) "I hate being in this room! Why can't I come out?" Discussed purpose of isolation; reassured concerning punishment. Janie talked on phone to other patients for 45 minutes
		(2) Refusal to take medicine	(2) Medical play	(2) "It tastes yukky!" Reinforced idea that medicine would help her get well and go home.

nation are also contained in this section.

(3) *The laboratory section* contains the results of diagnostic tests ordered by the physician.

In hospitals using the Problem-Oriented Medical Record system (POMR), the information contained in the preceding three sections is termed the *data base*, or the information necessary to formulate a comprehensive care plan. Since the POMR system is based on the identification of medical, social, or emotional problems with planned interventions to reduce or eliminate those problems, the next component of a POMR chart is the *problem list*. The problems identified are prioritized and numbered, so that they can be referred to by the assigned number in other portions of the chart. Following the problem list is a section outlining the *care plan* for the patient, based upon the problems previous delineated.

Both traditional medical records systems and the POMR method contain a section for *progress notes*. Here members of the health care team record observations and interactions with patients, as well as their current assessments and recommendations for continued care. Separate sections may be maintained for physician's notes and those of other disciplines, or all may chart in the same section, depending on hospital policy.

A number of special reports may also be included in the patient's chart. Reports on consultation from specialists are contained in the chart, as are reports from the surgeon and anesthesiologist, if the patient had an operation.

Charting

When recording information in a patient chart, the child life worker must observe certain guidelines to make the notations understandable and useful to others. Notations should be kept brief. If abbreviations are used, they should conform to an authorized hospital listing. One must also remember that the patient's medical record is a legal document, and therefore erasures are not permissible. If an error is made in notation, a single line should be drawn through the mistake. By proceeding in this manner, questions of tampering with the document can be avoided. The time of notation must be entered in the record and each entry signed.

A widely accepted form of chart notation is the SOAP format, an acronym for its components: *S*ubjective observations, *O*bjective observations, *A*ssessments, and *P*lans.

The problem as perceived by the patient or the patient's family is recorded under *subjective observations*. The speaker's own words are used for subjective notation. Thus, a child life worker might enter the following observations in patients' charts, based on the statements of children: "My Daddy's never gonna come back!" or "Tell 'em I'll be good if they don't give me another shot" or "The doctor said it wasn't going to hurt, but it did! I hate that doctor!" Similarly, a parent's observation that "My daughter refuses to let me out of her sight" may be recorded by the child life worker as a subjective notation.

Whatever observations health care personnel make through seeing, hearing, or feeling the patient, with or without the use of medical instruments, are recorded under *objective notations*. Medical personnel might, for example, record a patient's temperature, a successful bowel movement, or that a patient walked for the first time post-surgically. Statements concerning a patient's observable behavior should be included in this section, without drawing conclusions based on those observations. Thus, the child life worker might note that a child repeatedly jabbed a doll in the forehead with a syringe while playing doctor, cried for ten minutes after her parents left, or trembled while watching another child start an IV on a doll.

Conclusions drawn by the health care worker from the subjective and objective observations are recorded in the *assessment section*. A child life worker may have made the subjective notation that a child playing doctor with a doll said, "She's been bad! I gotta give her a shot, and her mother can't help her." In addition, the child's mother said, "I generally leave the room when it's time for her blood work. I feel it's easier for everyone that way." Objective observations recorded in the chart were that the child grew tense, cried, and hid under a table when a laboratory worker entered. Based on these observations, the child life worker might make an *assessment* that the child is frightened of needles, fearing them as punishment, with that fear compounded by mother's absence during the procedures.

In the final section of the medical record note, the observer enters a *plan*, or course of action designed to alleviate the problem noted. The plan should be written in behavioral terms, stating specific actions to be taken. The child life worker who made the observations noted above concerning a child's response to needles might plan additional needle play sessions, arrange for the presence of mother during blood tests, and contact laboratory personnel to offer explanations and reassurance prior to any procedure. The entire entry in the patient's chart would appear in this fashion:

Date	*Time*	
6/28	1410	*S*: Playing doctor in the playroom with doll, "She's been bad! I gotta give her a shot, and her mother can't help her."
		Mother observing the play, "I generally leave the room when it's time for her blood work. I feel it's easier for everyone that way."
		O: Patient's eyes widened, muscles tightened when med. tech. entered playroom. Began crying and hid under table. Mother tried to coax her out.
		A: Needles are feared, viewed as punishment. Mother's

absence denies patient support during blood drawings, increasing patient's fear.

P: (1) Notify lab personnel of situation. Request they offer reassurance and explanations to mother and child prior to any procedure.

(2) Have mother present for all needle work.

(3) Continue needle play sessions for further assessment of problem and reassurance

B. Blodgett, *Child Life*

The "Kardex®"

In most hospitals a nursing care plan for each patient is recorded on a set of cards kept at the nurses' station of the unit. This source of information, commonly referred to as the "Kardex®" after the brand name of one type of card holder, is a valuable aid to the child life worker as a quick review of patient care. In addition to basic information such as name, age, room number, and diagnosis, the Kardex contains the child's dietary restrictions and permissible activity level, e.g. "bedrest," "up with assistance," "up in wheelchair," etc. Ready access to this information is essential in planning much of child life programming.

The basic goals and objectives for the patient are recorded on the card, as well as current problems in the patient's care and a brief description of interventions to meet the problems identified. Some of the problems identified by Nursing may require child life involvement. For example:

Problem	Intervention	Result
Patient withdrawn	Child Life to do puppet play.	Child smiled; talked briefly with the puppet.

In other cases the child life worker may identify a problem calling for nursing intervention. It is helpful to record this problem in the Kardex as well as the patient's chart to assure prompt action. For example:

Problem	Intervention	Result
Patient expresses fear of shadows in room at night.	Close closet door and leave night-light on.	Patient slept comfortably through the night.

Communication among hospital professionals is essential if a patient is to receive the best care possible. Insights that child life workers obtain through their close contact with child and family are valuable to all other professionals involved in patient care. Through participation in health care team conferences and through utilization of patient records and the Kardex, a continual flow of valuable information between child life and other professionals is assured.

Although a major emphasis of child life programming is placed on the cooperation among professionals, barriers frequently arise to inhibit this goal. As one of the newer members of the health care team, child life workers, for various reasons, may not be readily accepted as equal partners in the care of children. In the following section, sources of resistance to child life programming and various means of reducing it will be explored.

COPING WITH RESISTANCE TO CHILD LIFE PROGRAMMING

Because hospitals are such complex institutions and child life programs are relatively new, it is virtually inevitable that there will be opposition to the establishment, expansion or alteration of the child life program from other groups within the hospital.

This opposition is rarely the result of "personality conflicts." More often it emerges because the role and function of the child life worker may parallel or conflict with those of another group within the hospital system. By recognizing and evaluating potential sources of resistance early enough, one can intervene effectively before the resistance becomes entrenched.

Sources of Resistance

Although it is possible to pinpoint countless different reasons for resistance to a child life program, our experience has been that they generally fall into the following eleven types:

IMPLIED CRITICISM OF OTHER STAFF. The child life program may be viewed by one or more other groups as pointing up their inadequacies. Otherwise, why would a child life program be necessary?

TERRITORIALITY. The child life program is sometimes seen as impinging on the domain of another program or service.

JEALOUSY. Others may envy the child life worker, particularly the special attention paid the new program or the warm response the child life worker usually gets from children and parents.

APATHY. Others may lack the interest or energy to support the goals of child life.

PERCEIVED MEDICAL AND/OR EMOTIONAL NEEDS. Others may differ in their assessments of what is best for the child.

FINANCIAL CONSIDERATIONS. Limited resources must be shared by many departments and personnel. The resources that support the child life program must be in some sense "taken away from" some other group.

RESPONSIBILITY TO SUPERIORS. Others may be concerned about the way their actions with respect to the child life program will be viewed by their superiors.

NEED TO MAINTAIN CONTROL. Many persons are strongly motivated by a need to manage and control, and they view anything they cannot directly control as a threat.

STATUS/TRAINING CONCERNS. Others may ascribe lower status to the child life worker or worry that the child life worker may not have appropriate training.

JOB SECURITY. Others may see the child life program as threatening their jobs.

PERSONAL INCONVENIENCE. Approval of the child life program may require others to work harder or at least change their work routines.

Not all these sources of resistance are likely to apply to every group within the hospital system. For each group, different reasons for resistance are more dominant.

Hospital Administration

Perhaps the most serious source of resistance among administrators is concern about finances. The child life program, by its very nature, does not generate clearly identifiable revenues for the hospital. An administrator may feel that the program is too expensive to justify, particularly since the costs cannot readily be charged to patients or third-party payers. With inflation putting increased strain on the hospital budget and consumers clamoring for lower health care costs, administrators are often reluctant to support the establishment or expansion of a child life program. Even when it appears the funds might be available, there is frequently intense pressure from other departments in the hospital, who feel they have greater need for the money. If the administrator is not convinced of the inherent value of the child life program, it may be easier to give funds to other departments, rather than risk their ire by funding child life.

Another source of resistance among administrators is the need to control and pass judgement. They may be unwilling to approve any change until all questions have been answered to their satisfaction, so that they can have a sense of control over what is happening within the organization they head. They want to know, for example, what changes in policy will be necessary, what other personnel will be affected, what the long-range implications will be, what demands for resources will be placed on various departments, and so forth. Raising questions about these matters does not mean that an administrator fails to perceive the merits of the program. It means only that the administrator wants to be "on top of" what is happening in the hospital.

Administrators also resist child life programs because they worry about what their superiors might think if they give the program their support. Approval of a program change might displease those to whom the administrator is responsible, such as the medical staff or the board of directors. Despite what health care personnel sometimes think, hospital administrators do not have the "last word." They too have superiors who expect certain things of them, and often they are very vulnerable to the actions of a displeased board of directors or medical director.

Often a change is resisted by administrators because of their differing views of the medical and/or emotional needs of children. The administrator may think, for example, that increased visitation by parents will endanger children's health and is emotionally upsetting, or that carpeting for the playroom cannot be purchased because it is a health hazard. Sometimes these views are based on good evidence; other times, not. But in all cases they are the legitimate perceptions of the administrator about what is best for the children the hospital serves.

Finally, apathy can explain the resistance of some administrators. They may have so many concerns demanding their attention that they simply are not interested in one more program to be responsible for. Or they may admit that there is value in the child life program, but simply not consider it a priority.

Medical Staff

Among the reasons why a child life program may be resisted by medical staff is the need to control. Physicians often see themselves as ultimately responsible for the care patients receive and want to control access to the patient. Although in some hospitals the trend toward a multidisciplinary team approach to patient care has eroded the view of the physician as the person controlling all decisions related to patients, most hospitals still operate with a fairly strict hierarchical structure.

The medical staff may also have a different perception of the patients' emotional and medical needs from that of child life workers. Physicians may consider parental presence upsetting to children, may not think children need special facilities for play, or may even disagree that hospitalization poses any threat to a child's psychological well-being. Since physicians rarely have much training in child development and are generally more concerned about correcting physical problems than easing psychological distress, it is not surprising that their point of view on what is best for young patients may differ from that of the child life worker. This is not to say, however, that they are insensitive to the patient's needs. They merely look at those needs from another viewpoint.

Sometimes the medical staff may simply be apathetic when it comes to the child life program, considering it to be a nice frill, but little more. We know of numerous hospitals in which most physicians are not even aware of the existence of a child life program, since their contact with the patients is limited to brief contacts for examinations or treatment procedures.

Nursing Staff

Although in a great number of hospitals the nursing staff is the group which can be counted on most to support the goals of the child life program, nurses can nevertheless be a source of resistance. They may, for example, see the presence of the child life worker as an indication that nursing has not fulfilled its function of caring for the child (implied criticism). Similarly, nurses may feel that a portion of their responsibility has been usurped by the child life worker. This is a "territoriality" issue, and it is particularly acute in the case of nurses whose training has emphasized the importance of attending to the emotional needs of the patient.

Jealousy accounts for certain instances of resistance to the child life program by nurses. To the nurse who must unwillingly but inevitably inflict pain and discomfort on his or her young patient, who must debride burns, empty bedpans, and change messy dressings, it often appears that the child life worker does only the "fun" parts of the child's care. Since the role of the child life worker will probably provoke more positive emotional responses from children than will the nurse's, nurses may resent not being "rewarded" as generously for their efforts.

Another source of resistance among nurses may be personal inconvenience. Sometimes the nursing staff may be unwilling to make the changes in scheduling patient care needed for a successful child life program, or they may resist altering the physical environment of the ward —to facilitate parents' rooming-in, for example. In some cases, this unwillingness springs, not from an ideological disagreement with the child life program, but from the personal inconvenience it will cause the nurse.

Worries about the way their actions will be viewed by superiors also accounts for resistance by nurses. We are familiar with an instance in which staff nurses saw the benefits of wearing colorful smocks rather than the white uniforms required by hospital policy, but they were afraid to push for the change for fear of encountering the disapproval of the director of nursing. In another hospital, nurses hesitated to cooperate with the child life worker to implement a preparation program because they assumed it would be opposed by the chief of pediatric surgery.

As with administrators and medical staff, nurses can resist the establishment of a child life program because they have perceptions of the medical and emotional needs of children that differ from those of the child life worker. Although it is rarely the case, some nurses still question the value of a play program for sick children, for example. Others oppose allowing parents to be present during medical procedures, or they minimize the need for preoperative preparation. This results from an honest difference of opinion as to what constitutes good patient care.

Resistance to the child life program by nurses can also result from apathy. Considering their heavy workload, the multitude of duties they must perform, and the constant demands on them by patients and physicians alike, it is not surprising that nurses often have no interest in supporting another program.

Mental Health Services

Psychologists, psychiatrists, and social workers, although they share many of the same goals as the child life worker, may resist the establishment of a child life program. One reason is implied criticism. They interpret the presence of the child life worker as an indication that someone thinks that the mental health professionals are failing to serve children and families adequately. Although this perception may be inaccurate, it nevertheless accounts for some reluctance by the mental health service to support the child life program.

Similarly, territoriality issues are often involved where mental health professionals are concerned. The child life worker is seen as taking over part of their responsibilities, since they too have the child's emotional well-being as a primary concern and use many of the same intervention strategies as the child life worker.

Another source of resistance with this group is the question of job security. We know of one hospital in which a social worker asked, "Why should a child life program be funded while our existing social service department is understaffed?" This social worker sees jobs going to child life workers that otherwise might be filled by social workers.

Another concern that mental health professionals may have is that of status and training. They may wonder if the child life workers are properly trained for the roles they are taking. In one hospital, the staff psychologist opposed a rap group for adolescents conducted by the child life worker. The psychologist asked, "Should someone with only a B.A. be doing this? Is the child life worker performing counseling services for which she is not qualified?" In another hospital, the social work department raised questions about the parents group that the child life department instituted each afternoon at 4:00 P.M., on the grounds that the child life worker leading the discussions had not had a college course in how to conduct groups. Sometimes these status and training concerns are groundless; at other times they are justified. But in all cases, it is most helpful to view them as the legitimate perceptions of another group of professionals.

Volunteer Services

A sometimes overlooked source of resistance in some hospitals is the office or person who has responsibility for recruiting and orienting volunteers. They have been known to view the establishment of a child life program as implied criticism of their own efforts, particularly if volunteers have been used extensively in the pediatric unit. They may assume that hiring a child life worker means that volunteers have failed to serve children adequately.

Other issues causing concern for the volunteer office are those related to territoriality. If a child life program is instituted, it may be necessary to resolve who will supervise volunteers in pediatrics — the child life worker or the volunteer director. The volunteer director may also worry that the role of volunteers will be reduced because of the presence of the child life staff.

Occupational Therapy

Like other groups in the hospital, the occupational therapy department may view the establishment of a child life program as implying criticism of them. They may fear that others think they have not been doing their jobs adequately; otherwise, why would child life services be necessary?

Because the role of the child life worker seems to overlap somewhat that of the occupational therapist (indeed, it is not unheard of for the child life program to be housed in the occupational therapy department), territoriality concerns may also arise, with occupational therapists feeling that part of their roles have been taken over by the child life workers.

Similarly, job security also can become an issue, with OT's wondering why their department was not enlarged rather than adding this "new breed" of health care professional, the child life worker. Their resistance may also grow out of a concern over the status and training of the child life worker: does she or he have the training needed to perform the job adequately?

Jealousy, too, can cause other therapists to oppose the child life program. Most OT's must work within fairly strict time schedules, seeing patients only for limited periods of time and within the somewhat artificial context of the treatment session. They may be jealous of the child life worker's opportunity to have prolonged contact with young patients and to interact with them in a more natural, spontaneous way.

It would be easy to assume from the foregoing discussion of the sources of resistance that the authors are implying that all of the members of all of these groups are likely to display resistance for all of the reasons mentioned. Of course, that is not true. Countless administrators can be depended on for solid support of child life. In numerous hospitals the impetus for establishing a child life program has come from the medical staff. Nurses are often the most supportive group in the hospital. Social workers, psychologists, psychiatrists, occupational therapists, and volunteer directors are all potential allies of the child life staff.

What the authors *are* saying, though, is that when resistance is encountered, there may be one or more reasons for it, growing out of the fact that the hospital is a system of interrelated groups. The first step in dealing with that resistance must necessarily be assessing its possible sources, and the types of resistance discussed above are a good place to begin.

Possible Interventions

When you are aware of the possible sources of resistance in a particular group, it is more effective to keep it from developing rather than to wait until you have to try to counteract it. Or to use a cliché, "An ounce of prevention is worth a pound of cure." If you can anticipate the possibility of resistance and can act to head it off, the results will be much more satisfactory than if you wait until you have to struggle to overcome resistance that has gathered strength and momentum. Three approaches may be considered:

(1) Education,

(2) Reassurance, and

(3) Offering services that meet the needs of members of the resistant groups.

Education

Education helps to counter almost all the types of resistance discussed previously. The most obvious form an educational intervention can take is the formal inservice. For example, for a hospital in which a child life program has only recently been established or in which the staff is poorly informed about the program, you might wish to offer an inservice on "The Role of the Child Life Worker." Assuming that the nursing staff was the identified area of potential resistance, you might wish to utilize an inservice design such as the following:

Part I: Effects of Hospitalization on Children and Families
  Material discussed:
  1. Characteristic problems various age-groups experience during hospitalization
  2. Effects of a child's hospitalization on parents and siblings
  Purpose: To establish that problems and needs exist
  Sources of resistance countered: Apathy, differences in perceived medical and/or emotional needs.

Part II: Possible Solutions
  Material discussed:
  1. Environmental changes—reinforce staff for changes that have already occurred and suggest others
  2. Changes in play and preparation procedures
  Purpose: To show staff that alternatives to present practices are available
  Sources of resistance countered: Differences in perceived medical and/or emotional needs, responsibility to superiors (nurses are given reasons why changes are necessary and should be pursued)

Part III: Who Should Do This?
  Material Discussed:
  1. Problems with present hospital situation
    a. Nurses lack time; medical needs are a priority
    b. Volunteers lack time and training
    c. Other services are already overburdened or lack proper training.
  2. Child life worker may be useful in meeting the important needs of

the hospitalized child and family which present staff are prevented from meeting.

Purpose: To show that the present staff have too many demands on their time to institute the desirable changes identified earlier.

Sources of resistance countered: Implied criticism, territoriality.

Other formal opportunities can be utilized to convey to the other persons in the hospital what the child life worker does and why these services are needed. One of the authors had success with a day-long "open house" in the playroom (announced several days in advance through posters and the hospital newsletter), during which hospital staff had a chance to examine play equipment, materials used for preparation, and audiovisual materials with which they might not have been familiar.

Educational interventions need not always be so formal and carefully organized. Informal contacts and casual conversations with members of the resistant groups, in which you attempt to explain what you do and why you do it, can often be just as effective. Brief articles about the goals and activities of the child life program can be inserted in the hospital newsletter from time to time with good results.

Reassurance

Reassurance is somewhat similar to education as an intervention strategy, but it focuses on the particular form of resistance you have perceived. For example, if you sense that other professionals in the hospital are resisting because of status/training concerns, you may wish to make sure that you communicate to them the preparedness of the child life worker — particularly that the child life worker knows the importance of the program, that he or she has a thorough knowledge of the literature concerning hospitalized children, and that he or she has the proper vision of the program that is being established. At the same time, it is essential to guard against giving others the impression that child life "knows it all" or "has all the answers." Arrogance and throwing one's weight around will not only fail to reassure others, but will inevitably create increased resistance.

Another form of reassurance is cooperation. Rather than viewing your program as being the sole source of emotional support for patients, you should try to facilitate the functioning of the various disciplines as a unified health care team. Of course, there is little you can do to compel others to accept you as a team member, but you can do much to treat others as your colleagues in meeting the needs of children. This will go far in dispelling their fears that you are there because they are not doing their jobs well or because you seek to take their jobs away from them.

In trying to reassure others of your competence and of the value of the child life program, it is helpful to bring off some early successes. Select an initial goal that is readily attainable, so that others see you as able to do something well. Your initial goal, besides being readily *attainable* (to assure you of early success), should also be one that is *important to your program objectives* (so that you are not wasting your time on something trivial), *visible* to other staff members (so that your efforts do not go unnoticed), and *welcomed* by the staff (so that they are glad you have accomplished it).

For example, in going into a hospital that had not previously had a child life program, the authors found that refurbishing a dreary, poorly equipped playroom was a good way to begin. With a minimal financial investment and relatively little effort, we were able to give the hospital personnel tangible evidence of what a child life program could mean to them. In addition, since the medical staff held their weekly meetings in that same room, the attending pediatricians were confronted very quickly with visible proof that we were accomplishing something.

For persons who are resistant because they fear the way their actions will be viewed by a superior, your reassurance may need to include smoothing the way with their superior. If a head nurse is reluctant to change a policy because he or she fears the reaction of the director of nursing, but shows no inclination of asking the director for his or her opinion, it may be helpful for you to approach the director of nursing directly and then return to the head nurse with the necessary reassurance of that person's approval.

Offering Services

Offering services that meet the needs of members of resistant groups is another useful approach. That is, others will be less threatened, and hence less resistant, if they can see that the child life program benefits them personally or makes their jobs easier or gives them recognition and esteem. For the administration, the child life program offers an improved image of the hospital, the possibility of attracting an increased number of patients, and praise from patients and parents pleased with the services offered.

For both the medical staff and the nursing staff, the child life program can provide increased cooperation on the part of patients, a shortened period of recuperation, and increased understanding of the child's emotional state. The authors know of at least one hospital where surgeons now refuse to operate on children who have not been prepared by the child life worker and where the operating room nurses speak enthusiastically about how much more pleasant their jobs are now that they no longer have to forcibly restrain terror-stricken young patients while anesthesia is administered.

The child life worker can enhance the social work department by identifying and referring new clients who might previously have been missed and by providing additional information on patients, through observations of play and of parent-child interaction.

The child life program similarly meets the needs of the volunteer coordinator by providing interesting and valuable experiences for volunteers and identifying new areas where volunteers can be utilized, such as preadmission tours and special play sessions. If the child life worker must train and supervise volunteers for a specific project, the volunteer coordinator should be consulted regularly to assure that the coordinator maintains appropriate control over the activities of volunteers.

The needs of occupational therapy can be met by identifying patients that need their services and by providing follow-up on their recommendations through child life activities. Often OT's feel isolated from participation in the total care of the child, since their contact is usually strictly scheduled into certain time slots each day or week. The child life worker can draw these persons into a spirit of teamwork by offering to provide continuity between the therapy session and the child's life on the ward.

None of these interventions guarantee you instantaneous or unlimited support and approval of others within the hospital system. Such unqualified support is unrealistic to expect. But by attempting to identify and methodically counter the most apparent sources of resistance before they have an opportunity to become entrenched, you are likely to encounter fewer obstacles in the introduction and expansion of child life services.

CHAPTER 9

SUPERVISION OF VOLUNTEERS, STUDENTS, AND STAFF

EXTENDING SERVICES WITH AUXILIARY PERSONNEL

The task of providing sensitive care to hospitalized children and their families often appears to be herculean. As one problem is identified and traced back to its source, several other concerns arise, demanding intervention from the child life worker. For example, as an attempt is made to relieve the boredom of children through the dissemination of play materials, an undercurrent of anxiety is still apparent in their play. The keen observer of the activity of children finds the continual emergence of common themes: aggression, separation, protection, and control. Following play of this sort, the anxiety of children seems to subside. In response, the child life worker expands the emphasis of the play program to provide more opportunities for self-expression and for mastery of the difficult elements of hospitalization through play media.

And so the cycle continues. The themes emphasized through the play of children indicate the need for change in the services and practices of the hospital. For example, a properly functioning preparation program could dispel the misconceptions revealed by children in doctor play sessions. A program to encourage the presence of parents might lessen the fears of abandonment so frequently observed in doll play. Or an inservice for laboratory personnel on communication with young children could reduce the belief that needlework is a mechanism for punishing misdeeds.

To attempt the institution of any of these changes requires a tremendous commitment of time, a limited commodity in child life programming. Hopefully as new programming needs are identified and their value demonstrated (see Chapter 10), additional personnel will supplement the child life staff. Another means of extending the time available for the implementation of new services is through the use of volunteer workers or students, who may perform a portion of the child life tasks.

Whether additional help comes from paid hospital personnel or through the service of volunteers, the presence of subordinates thrusts the child life worker into a supervisory role, requiring the exercise of skills quite different from those previously employed. Due to the frequency with which child life workers are called upon to function in a supervisory capacity, it is important to consider such basic issues as the orienting of new personnel, maintaining the interest of volunteers in their duties, evaluating performance, and offering feedback to subordinates concerning their work.

THE USE OF VOLUNTEERS AND STUDENTS

As valuable as volunteers and students may be in achieving the goals of child life programming and expanding the range of available services, their contributions will not be realized unless the child life worker expends tremendous energy preparing for their presence. An orientation to the hospital facility and its procedures, as well as familiarization with play areas and materials, is needed. Those who have not previously worked with children will require an introduction to child development principles and the special concerns of children in each age-group when hospitalized. Schedules must be coordinated and their work supervised to foster their improvement and to assure the proper care of the children.

The burden of performing this function adequately may be too great for the child life worker attempting to establish a new program, actually resulting in a decrease of the total child life time available to patients. For this reason, it may be advisable for a new child life worker to delay the acceptance of volunteers and students until the basic elements of the program are better established, unless a substantial portion of the orientation and supervision can be performed by other personnel such as the director of volunteer services.

Volunteer Positions

Once the child life worker feels comfortable in accepting the responsibility for training and supervising volunteers, then the volunteers can be incorporated into the existing program in a variety of capacities:

Playroom Supervision

Volunteers may assist the child life worker in the supervision of playroom activities, perhaps conducting a specific activity or aiding small groups or individuals. The presence of a competent volunteer in the playroom offers the child life worker the flexibility to leave the area to pursue other projects or offer children individualized attention as needed. In addition to the supervision of children, playroom volunteers can assist in maintenance and clean-up, straightening cabinets, discarding broken toys, and noting supplies which need to be replenished.

Activities for Children in Rooms

At times the volume of children in the playroom, or the specialized type of activity offered in that location, will demand the presence of the child life worker. In such cases volunteer assistants may be used to visit children in their rooms who, because of their medical conditions, are unable to join in playroom activities.

Substitute Parents

Some volunteers, who are capable of donating large blocks of time and who have shown a particular affinity for the care of children, may be specially trained to serve as "substitute parents" or "foster grandparents." When a child's parents are unable to visit the hospital because of their work, the distances involved, or other reasons, the child can be assigned a volunteer parent who can, in the words of Hardgrove and Dawson (1972), "provide the child with an ongoing and personal relationship, a special friendship distinct from the nursing care (p. 235)."

Entertainment

The performing talents of other volunteers may be tapped to entertain children in their rooms, in impromptu hallway gatherings, or in more formal program settings. Singers, actors, musicians, jugglers, and others may visit regularly or provide entertainment on special occasions. (See Guidelines for Visiting Groups, Chapter 7.)

Use of Special Skills

Volunteers may possess special interests or skills that they particularly wish to share with children. The child life worker can maintain a file of interested stamp collectors, chess players, electricians, artisans, naturalists, and others who wish to share their time and knowledge with children of similar interests. When a child wishes to explore one of these areas, the appropriate volunteer can be contacted and arrangements made for a visit.

Supportive Services

Rather than directly applying skills in interaction with children, some volunteers may donate their time and efforts to enhance the play environment of the hospital. Members of a garden club, for example, may volunteer their energies to maintain the plantings of an outdoor play area. A woodworking group may provide durable, hand-crafted toys, while students in an industrial arts class perform major repair work on playroom equipment. Services of this type are of invaluable assistance in operating safe, attractive play areas on a limited source of funds. And since these volunteers have little direct contact with children, they generally require less orientation and supervision.

Family Assistance

Parents are often prevented from participating actively in the care of their hospitalized children by the practical restraints of limited transportation to the hospital or inability to find proper supervision for non-hospitalized siblings. A portion of the volunteer personnel may devote their efforts to providing services to assist in these situations. Volunteer drivers may call for parents at their homes, delivering them to the hospital and providing return transportation as needed.

Other volunteers may be recruited to supervise siblings in the hospital (if no sibling play area is presently staffed by the child life department), or they may stay with the nonhospitalized siblings in the family's home. According to Hardgrove (1972),

> Some volunteers may be more comfortable helping out at home rather than in the hospital. For most volunteers their previous experience would be more relevant in the home, and the children who are still well and in a familiar environment are better able to accept and enjoy the substitute mother than is the child in the hospital (p. 51).

Clerical Work

The precious time of the child life worker is often consumed by the writing of "thank you" notes and other correspondence, ordering of supplies, the clipping and filing of articles, and other important clerical tasks. Even when hospital clerical services are available to the child life staff, special projects invariably lie dormant, waiting for "another day." The efficiency of the child life staff in performing normal duties and in attempting new projects is greatly enhanced through the use of volunteer office assistance.

Assistance in Special Programming

The implementation of many worthy programs for children would have to be abandoned or delayed, due to lack of personnel, if it were not for the work of volunteers. For example, the task of calling parents prior to the admission of their children, inviting them to the preadmission tour, though effective in relieving parental anxiety and increasing participation in the tour, may be overwhelming for a single child life worker. Volunteers trained specifically for this purpose may complete the calls in a more thorough, unhurried manner. Similarly, the number of children participating in preadmission tours may necessitate the adoption by volunteers of a portion of the responsibilities. Trained volunteers can conduct tours of the hospital, assist children in play sessions, or supervise the dispensing of treats.

Seasoned members of the volunteer corps, knowledgeable of hospital routines and the needs of their fellow workers, may turn their efforts toward the development of orientation sessions for new volunteers. With the assistance of the child life worker and the director of volunteer services, these individuals can compile a volunteer handbook, conduct hospital tours highlighting areas of special importance to volunteer workers, and lead discussion groups designed to help the new workers cope with feelings elicited by the hospital environment.

Student Positions

In addition to the volunteer labor recruited from the community at large, child life workers may contact educational institutions to seek the participation of students. High school students may be asked to volunteer time after school, or may obtain released time to perform duties in conjunction with their classroom work. College students from education, child psychology, or social work programs are frequently required to donate a given number of hours in volunteer work, or they seek placements for practicum experiences. Working with hospitalized children is a unique field placement, likely to attract a number of qualified students knowledgeable in child development and interested in examining a potential career.

The type of work in which students will engage depends on their past educational experiences, personal level of maturity, and the requirements of their scholastic program. Generally, the role of student worker will be limited to direct involvement with small groups and individual children, as well as the maintenance and supervision of the playroom and materials. More specialized assignments such as making preadmission calls, serving as substitute parents, or organizing orientation sessions are better left to volunteers able to make a long-term commitment to serve. A student spending a semester in a child life program is more likely to benefit from exposure to a variety of activities which offer an overview of the services, rather than more intensive involvement in a narrow aspect of programming.

Students working in the hospital as a full-time practice experience will generally arrive with a set of expectations formulated by the scholastic program. Their requirements may be closely defined, calling for specific amounts of observation and participation in various activities, e.g. preoperative teaching, play with various ages, attendance at case conferences, etc. In other cases, the student's experiences will be left to the discretion of the supervisor, in consultation with the student. With either arrangement it is important to review the expectations of the student prior to the commencement of fieldwork to be certain that both the child life worker and the student agree on the content of the experience. It may be helpful to draft a contract describing the types of experiences offered to the student and including the expectations the child life worker has for the student's performance. If the child life worker will be required to evaluate the student's performance, specific criteria for assessment may be included in this document. The presence of these standards permits the student to perform periodic self-evaluations and further reduces the frequent complaint that assessments are overly subjective, based on ill-defined norms.

INTRODUCTION OF VOLUNTEERS AND STUDENTS TO THE HOSPITAL SETTING

The demand for child life services is often so great that the child life worker fortunate enough to locate volunteer or student help is tempted to orient them briefly and immediately press the workers into service. To present a more protracted orientation session is viewed as too time-consuming, given the pressure of other duties. However, the time saved through limiting the orientation process may represent false economy. A moderate amount of additional time and planning invested in the introduction of volunteers and students to their new duties will help the child life worker avoid the greater cost of frustration and wasted hours at a later date. Among common problems encountered by child life workers when using student or volunteer help are the following:

(1) After a brief orientation session and an initial taste of the job to be performed, the volunteer or student quits. This may be due to the individual's inability to cope with the medical environment, to differences between the worker's expectations and the reality of the situation, or merely to the person's confusion and feelings of incompetence.

(2) The bewildered, but conscientious new worker asks an endless stream of questions, taxing the time and patience of the child life worker.

(3) The confused, but less than conscientious new worker commits a series of mistakes, e.g. lifting children improperly, failing to note the volume of fluids consumed by children, walking into isolation rooms without taking the proper precautions, requiring the close supervision of the individual by the child life worker and, perhaps, ultimate dismissal.

(4) The individual's attendance becomes sporadic, and duties are performed without commitment. Eventually the person stops coming to the hospital, or, if a student in need of credit, retreats to minimal requirements.

Many of these problems can be reduced or eliminated if the child life worker adopts new procedures for accepting and training new volunteers and students. If the hospital employs a director of volunteer services, these measures can be established in consultation with that individual.

Preorientation Observation

Little is more frustrating for the time-conscious child life worker than to have a newly trained volunteer or student quit immediately after orientation. Equally annoying is the discovery that the individual who has received an orientation is unsuited to perform the duties requested and must be dismissed. In either case, valuable hours are lost, thereby tempting the child life worker to abandon the use of volunteers or severely limit the time spent in training. Problems of this nature often arise because the prospective volunteer has been unable to gain a realistic picture of the work situation or because the child life worker has had limited opportunity to assess the potential of the individual to function in the hospital setting. A prospective volunteer or student may, for example, have passed through an initial screening interview with the volunteer director or child life worker while holding the mistaken belief that a "play person" does little more than read books to bed-fast children. When confronted with the reality of the pediatric unit, the volunteer may be shocked at the active, frequently aggressive nature of the children and may be offended when few will gather around for "story time." Other newcomers may have underestimated their emotional reaction to the medical setting, finding it impossible to function amid the suffering of children.

Similarly, the child life worker, who has had only limited contact with the prospective worker prior to orientation, may have difficulty gauging the suitability of the volunteer to work with children under potentially stressful conditions. The individual who appears quite calm and competent in the more relaxed setting of an office interview may behave quite differently in a noisy playroom with active children underfoot.

To avoid problems such as these, the child life worker may require the prospective volunteer or student to spend a period of time observing child life activities before a decision is made to accept the individual for orientation. The period of observation should correspond in length and time of day to the shift the volunteer is likely to work. This allows the individual to view a variety of activities and to judge the pattern of occurrences likely to be encountered during regular service. While the prospective volunteer or student has an opportunity to experience the medical setting and watch the interactions of child life workers and children, the child life worker is also permitted an extended chance to view the person's responses.

Following the observation period, the prospective volunteer and child life worker meet again to discuss their responses to the situation. If the mutual reaction to the observation period is positive, arrangements can be made for formal orientation as a child life volunteer. Based on the period of observation, however, some potential workers may decide that their initial impulses to spend time in the hospital were misguided. These individuals may withdraw from the program prior to orientation having made minimal demands on the child life worker's time.

At times individuals whom after the observation period the child life worker believes to be unsuited to work with children may wish to pursue the orientation sessions. In such cases the child life worker may attempt to counsel the person into another branch of volunteer service more appropriate to his or her talents and personality. If the individual refuses to consider an alternate assignment, it may be necessary to eliminate this person from further consideration as a volunteer.

The Orientation Period

Many new volunteers and students enter the program having had limited previous experience with children or medical care settings. During the period of orientation it will therefore be necessary to familiarize participants with hospital geography and relevant policies and procedures. A review of the normal development of children and their common response when under stress is also in order. In addition to this knowledge, skills necessary for interaction with children and their parents should be discussed and practiced. Finally, a discussion of common problems encountered and typical personal reactions of volunteers to their work will help the new recruits in their adjustment to the new role.

Familiarization with the Medical Setting

Naturally, new workers will need a tour of the facility, covering not only their immediate work area, but all major locations also. This eases their comfort in the new surroundings and gives them a better understanding of the various areas of the hospital serving children. Important landmarks within the assigned working area should be emphasized. If working in the pediatric unit, for example, the nurses' station, kitchen, bathrooms, and storage facilities should be identified. Volunteers and students should also be familiar with patient rooms, learning the mysteries of lowering siderails, raising beds, locking wheelchair wheels, and calling for the nurse. Particular attention should be devoted to the play facilities, familiarizing the new workers with the range of available materials and the means of locating them.

In addition to the physical surroundings, new volunteers and students must be aware of basic hospital policies, should the need to implement them arise. New workers must be familiar with the hospital fire and disaster plans and the role they will be expected to play should these events occur. It is also wise to show trainees the location of fire extinguishers in the pediatric unit, and review the types of fires on which each is used.

Of more immediate concern to the new volunteers and students is an understanding of the hospital's infection control policies. Individuals should be taught to recognize isolation rooms and how to respond to the various types of isolation. Despite a review of this material, new workers should be told to refrain from entering these rooms without consulting hospital staff, until they are fully comfortable with all procedures. The child life worker should also discuss the limitations on the types of materials which may enter children's rooms, based on the infection precautions in effect.

Finally, new volunteers and students should be aware of the actions they should take in the event of a seizure or other medical emergency. In the case of a seizure, the volunteer should attempt to protect the patient from injury, while not restraining him or her. Immediate medical attention should be sought, but the patient should not be left alone. Observations made by the volunteer should be reported to medical personnel, as they may be helpful in diagnosis or treatment of the child's condition.

Familiarization with Child Development

Since their working knowledge of childhood may be limited, new volunteers and students should be informed of the common behaviors and capacities of children of various ages. Examples of activities successful with each age-group may be demonstrated and the benefits of these related to the developmental level of the children. An effort should be made to transmit an appreciation of the value of play to children in general and hospitalized children in particular. The importance of play in allowing children to master the difficult and in enhancing self-expression should therefore be emphasized.

Volunteers and students will doubtlessly observe much in their play and interaction with children of value to the child life workers and other members of the health care team. The hidden anger of a child revealed through a doll play session, the candid expression of a personal fear, or the hesitancy of a patient to participate in playroom activities may indicate the need for further intervention. To be certain that this valuable information is not lost, trainees should receive practice in the observation of children and should be aware of proper methods of relaying this material.

Familiarization with Program Goals

The objectives of child life programming should be clearly presented to the new volunteers and students, so that they may more accurately see how the efforts requested of them will fit into the total program. In addition, the expectations for the individual volunteer or student assignments should be clarified. These "job descriptions" should be specific enough to provide security for individuals troubled by ambiguous, ill-defined tasks, while not being so narrow as to inhibit the creativity and personal style through which each can enrich a program.

Guidelines for Performing Duties

Many of the problems commonly observed in the work of new volunteers and students can be avoided by the provision of an outline of basic rules of conduct. These guidelines, based on the necessities of the hospital setting and a knowledge of the needs of hospitalized children, may cover subjects such as hospital protocol, communication with children, and playroom management. Among the advice and expectations typically presented to newcomers are the following:

MAINTAIN CONFIDENTIALITY. During their period of hospital service, volunteers and students may become privy to information about the medical and emotional conditions of children and their families. All hospital workers must treat this knowledge as confidential, avoiding discussion of it outside the hospital.

ASCERTAIN THE CHILD'S CONDITION BEFORE FEEDING OR MOVING. Pediatric patients may ask for the assistance of volunteers or students in obtaining water or treats from the kitchen, using bathroom facilities, repositioning themselves in bed, or going for walks. Before agreeing to move patients or get refreshments for them, workers should check with the nursing staff to be certain that their actions are not inconsistent with the patient's medical care. Nurses should also be notified when children need to use the bathroom, as it may be necessary to measure the patient's output, examine the stool, or obtain a specimen.

HELP CHILDREN ONLY WHEN NEEDED. Many volunteers and students, new to the medical setting, may be overwhelmed with anger and sympathy upon viewing the condition of hospitalized children. Frustrated by their inability to do more to relieve the fears and pain of the children, some may attempt to compensate by acting toward children in an oversolicitous manner, performing functions such as feeding and dressing them, or retrieving their playthings that the children are capable of doing themselves. New workers must realize that this behavior encourages regression and passivity among patients, compounding the difficulty of their situation. Volunteers and students should, instead, be urged to explore the capacities of the children, helping to maintain and develop them while in the hospital.

APPROACH CHILDREN GENTLY. Children will be wary of strangers, especially while in the threatening environment of the hospital. Rapid, aggressive movement will nonverbally communicate danger to the child, thereby impeding efforts to initiate friendship. Children should be approached confidently, yet with gentleness, allowing them to accept the presence of a stranger as a benign individual. Preschoolers will be more receptive to the introduction of new people if approached in the presence of parents.

SPEAK SOFTLY. The tone of a person's voice is as important in communicating with a young child as the content of the words spoken. Volunteers and students should therefore attempt to address children in a soft, well-modulated manner, conveying a feeling of warmth and security.

BEND DOWN TO THE CHILD'S LEVEL. Despite the gentleness of a volunteer's approach and a kind, accepting manner of speech, children may still be intimidated by a stranger's presence, especially if the unfamiliar figure looms far overhead. New volunteers and students should be reminded to bend down to the child's level — better yet, to squat down so that one's head is on the same level as the child's. By doing so the worker reduces the threat engendered by physical height and facilitates the communication process with the child.

AVOID MAKING PROMISES THAT MAY NOT BE KEPT. Having started a friendship with a hospitalized child, the new volunteer or student may be tempted to solidify the new bonds by assenting to the child's request, even though the ability to fulfill the wish may not lie totally within the worker's power. The worker may promise to visit later in the day, participate in a desired activity, or accompany the child to an outdoor play area. Circumstances may change, however, causing the promise to be broken, albeit unintentionally. The child may be sleeping when the volunteer returns, the desired materials may be missing, or uncooperative weather may spoil the outing. To avoid unnecessary disappointment for children and a corresponding loss of faith in adults who fail to keep their word, volunteers and students should be counselled against making definite promises to children.

DO NOT OFFER CHILDREN ILLUSORY CHOICES. If a volunteer or student must leave a child to attend to another duty or if an activity must be temporarily interrupted for a medical treatment or examination, the child should be truthfully informed of the situation. Phrases such as, "Is it all right if we stop now?" or "We have to stop playing for a minute, okay?" are unfair to children, since they offer an apparent choice where none exists. New workers should be advised to eliminate these illusory choices from their communication with children.

BE POSITIVE WITH CHILDREN. The behavior problems that volunteers and students will encounter can be minimized if a consistent, positive approach to dealing with children is adopted. Children respond well to praise of their efforts, and workers should be ready to commend the desirable actions they exhibit.

When limitations must be placed on the activities of children, these, too, should be phrased positively, not merely proscribing an unacceptable behavior, but offering an alternative action. For example, rather than saying, "Don't play ball in the playroom!", one might say, "It's crowded here in the playroom. Let's bounce the ball in the hallway." Thus the child is offered an alternative acceptable behavior to replace that which is discouraged.

EXPLAIN THE REASONS BEHIND LIMITATIONS. In the preceding example, the child was offered a brief explanation of the need to change the location for playing ball—the playroom was too crowded. Whenever limitations are placed on behavior, children should be offered a similar explanation to avoid the belief that limitations are arbitrarily imposed by adults as a means of punishment. For example, if several children are actively, and noisily, involved in play in a room where another patient is asleep, the play should not be summarily squelched with the admonition, "Stop making that noise!" Instead, another location for play should be suggested, with an explanation of the sleeping patient's need for rest.

BE AWARE OF THE NEEDS OF ALL CHILDREN. The temptation exists for playroom workers to become highly involved with the activities of a single child or small group, to the exclusion of others in the area. This is especially true for new workers, who are seeking the security of a relationship and a structured activity in the unaccustomed surroundings. Playroom supervisors must be aware of the needs of all children in the area, seeing that they are involved in meaningful activities and facilitating the interaction among children. Recognizing that new volunteers and students may be uncomfortable in the playroom, the child life worker should initially limit their duties, allowing them a chance to adjust to the playroom environment before accepting major responsibility. When they are ready to assume a larger role in playroom affairs, the workers should be prepared to serve the needs of all children present.

HAVE SEVERAL ACTIVITIES READY. As new volunteers and students will soon discover, the attention span of many children is brief. After a limited exploration of one activity, the child's fascination for it may dwindle, as the anxious child girds for a new adventure. The new worker who has expected fingerpaints or playdough to satisfy the gang for an entire morning may be uncomfortably caught with few alternatives to offer. By having the materials for several back-up activities at hand, the playroom supervisor is better equipped to meet the demands of children's shifting interests.

ALLOW CHOICES IN THE ACTIVITIES. Children should be able to choose among several different activities. For those not drawn to the structured activities provided by the playroom supervisor, other forms of play should be readily available. New volunteers and students must be made aware of the importance of allowing hospitalized children to exercise choice and assert control in the playroom, since the opportunity to do so elsewhere in the hospital is so severely restricted.

DO NOT BE CONCERNED ABOUT MESSINESS. Active children, intensely involved in their play, will frequently tip over a pot of paint or dribble glue on the playroom floor. When these "accidents" occur, the playroom supervisor should tend to them with little fuss and avoid making the child feel to blame. Volunteers and students should be shown that the emphasis is placed on prevention of these mishaps, by placing paint in stable containers, providing smocks for the children and working on washable surfaces. Yet when the inevitable occurs, they should handle the situation calmly, and avoid comments that children could interpret as scolding.

ENCOURAGE PARENT PARTICIPATION. Among the goals of child life programming presented to the new volunteers and students during the orientation period is the facilitation of the parent-child relationship during hospitalization. As playroom supervisors, students and volunteers can aid in the advancement of this goal by encouraging parents to participate in playroom activities with their children. Parents may, however, wish to use the child's time in the playroom as an opportunity for a much-needed break. If this is the case, playroom supervisors should, of course, respect their wishes, welcoming the parents upon their return to the play area.

PREPARE CHILDREN FOR THE END OF ACTIVITIES. As lunchtime approaches, bedtime draws near or playroom activities must end for another reason, the playroom supervisor should advise the children, thereby allowing them to bring their play to a close. For example, the worker might prepare children by saying, "It's almost time for lunch. We can each take one more turn, then we must clean up." Students and volunteers should again be cautioned about offering children what seems like a choice in the matter ("Do you want to stop now? It's time to close the playroom.") if none exists.

KEEP CABINETS LOCKED. When in a hurry to dispense new materials to waiting children or to return children to their rooms following a play session, the playroom supervisor may accidentally forget to secure cabinets containing potentially hazardous materials. New students and volunteers should be reminded of the importance of locking all storage areas that contain paints, scissors, or other art materials or any toys or games containing small parts easily swallowed by young children. Failure to do so may result in disaster when one's attention is distracted for a brief period.

Anticipated Reactions

After familiarizing trainees with the hospital setting, child life programming, and their role within this milieu, some attention should be given to the feelings and reactions participants are likely to have when they commence their duties. Certain reactions are easily anticipated. Most new students and volunteers feel somewhat ill at ease in their attempts to locate necessary materials, initiate conversations with strangers, and mediate differences between children. Many feel anger and frustration as they view the suffering of children or immeasurable gratification as they receive a "thank you" from an appreciative parent. Some new workers, because of their own previous experiences in the medical setting, may feel discomfort as they step into their new roles.

The apprehensions new volunteers and students harbor may be reduced if they have an opportunity to discuss their feelings with others. Particularly helpful will be the insights of experienced workers, who may have shared the feelings of the new trainees yet found that, with time, these feelings diminished or were overshadowed by the pleasures of the work. The new recruit who feels awkward in approaching children gains comfort from the fact that others, now successful in their work, began in the same faltering way.

Maximizing the Effects of Orientation

The tremendous volume of material that must be presented to volunteers and students if they are to perform their duties effectively creates an obvious problem for the child life worker or volunteer director who must prepare an orientation: that is, how to transmit this material in a meaningful form, without overwhelming the participants. Among the possible solutions to this dilemma are the following techniques:

Variation of Activities

When preparing orientation activities, it is wise to minimize the use of the lecture format. While the oral presentation is an efficient mechanism for dispensing a large amount of information, an endless series of speakers and topics is likely to leave participants bored, tired and, perhaps worst, confused about the content of the material presented. In addition to having these shortcomings, the lecture format is also inadequate, since it frequently assumes a high degree of prior knowledge and experience from the listeners. The information presented by a speaker on the topic of playroom management, for example, will be of little benefit to an audience that has had limited contact with the playroom environment and is unacquainted with the normal behavior of children.

As an alternative, the orientation of new volunteers and students should provide for the *active involvement* of participants and supply a sampling of experiences that may be missing from their backgrounds. *Audiovisual aids* are extremely useful in several portions of the training process. For example, *videotape presentations* showing the normal play of children and their reactions to the hospital setting are more effective in preparing trainees for their future experiences than an oral exposition of the same subject matter. Similarly, audio- or videotape recordings of child life workers implementing the suggested guidelines for communicating with children provide a role model for participants, thereby delivering the material in a more meaningful way than through a mere recitation of the outline.

A variety of other visual aids may be used in the orientation. One of a number of excellent *films* depicting the reactions of children to hospitalization might be used to sensitize trainees to the difficulties encountered by young patients. *Photographic slides* showing the variety of activities available to children or describing special equipment for use with patients may be employed. Comments of other volunteers or students concerning their initial reactions to hospital work may be presented through *audio tape recordings*.

Much of the information to be presented during orientation lends itself nicely to the participation of trainees in *role play activities*. For example, participants may form small groups and practice the communication guidelines suggested earlier in this chapter, alternating turns in a child or an adult role. Simulated playroom situations can be presented, with trainees playing through the reactions of their assigned roles.

To vary the pace of orientation events and to reduce the uneasiness some volunteers and students may have with involvement in children's activities, *actual play materials* may be available. The opportunity for trainees to mix a batch of fingerpaints or test the properties of "home-made" modeling compound will increase their confidence once in the playroom setting and will add the important element of playfulness to the preservice training sessions.

Finally, events which *reinforce previous information* are valuable in increasing understanding and the retention of knowledge among partici-pants. For example, following the presentation of a movie depicting the reactions of children to hospitalization, trainees might discuss the extent to which personnel in the film followed the previously considered guide-lines for communication or playroom management. Azarnoff and Flegal (1975) suggest the use of "scavenger hunts," in which participants are asked to locate important hospital areas or personnel or discover the answers to key questions, as a possible means of reinforcing information learned in previous sessions.

Offering Limited Information during Initial Orientation Sessions

An alternative method of making the mass of material to be covered more comprehensible to trainees is to severely limit initial presentations, supplementing them with more complete information at a later time. The advantage of this method is that it allows students and volunteers to absorb information gradually, combining their work experiences with the addition of new and meaningful knowledge. For example, volunteers may be given a tour of the pediatric unit and play facilities before being assigned to work with a single child in the playroom. After volunteers have grown accustomed to the playroom environment, and have had an opportunity to observe the work of others, the staff may then make a more thorough presentation on playroom activities and management skills. Similarly, an initial orientation session may merely introduce the concept of patient isolation, enabling participants to recognize isolation rooms to avoid mistakenly entered them. At a later date the various forms of isolation techniques can be covered in greater depth.

Volunteer or Student Handbook

Whatever method of orienting new students and volunteers is chosen (either several intensive sessions at the beginning of service or a less comprehensive initial orientation followed by supplementary experiences), it is helpful to provide trainees with a handbook containing the informa-tion covered during this period. Despite the best efforts of child life personnel and volunteer services directors to present all information in a clear, accessible manner, it is inevitable that a portion of the material will be misunderstood or forgotten. Many questions that will undoubtedly arise during the course of a student or volunteer's service may be quickly answered by referring to the handbook.

Providing Support for Volunteers and Students

As mentioned previously, a student or volunteer's introduction to hospital work will likely be accompanied by a variety of conflicting feelings. The consideration of these feelings should not be disregarded upon the conclusion of orientation. Valuable volunteers who have not been afforded the opportunity to air their frustrations or resolve nagging conflicts will likely be lost from service to the program. For similar reasons, students may redirect their career objectives. To assure that students and volunteers have an adequate opportunity to express the feelings arising from their work and to receive corresponding support, the following measures may be implemented:

Regularly Scheduled Meetings with Supervisor

The child life worker supervising students or volunteers should hold periodic meetings with individual workers or with the group as a whole to explore their perceptions of the experience. These meetings may be run as an "open forum," or may concentrate on the specific concern identified by participants, e.g., the motivation behind a child's behavior, the use of play to help particular children, means of coping with one's feelings of helplessness.

The child life worker should be prepared for volunteers or students to challenge various elements of the program. Constructive criticism should be welcomed as an opportunity to review existing policies and methods of operating. Questions posed by students or volunteers may at times spring from their inexperience or their failure to observe certain conditions in the environment. The unworkable nature of a student's suggestion that playroom cabinets be left open for children to serve themselves, for example, can be easily answered by recounting tales of past "catastrophies." In other cases, however, the fresh insight of new workers will enable them to discover conditions requiring change or to conceive of preferable means of approaching a task.

Meetings of this type not only benefit new students and volunteers, by providing a forum for venting their feelings and expressing concerns, but also help the child life worker gain a better understanding of the needs of new personnel. Through a series of these discussions, the child life worker can determine the value of the information provided during the orientation process and may elicit suggestions for its improvement.

Support Groups

Volunteers and students may feel the need for additional support, which can be provided through the formation of independent discussion groups. Membership can be open to any volunteers and students who can meet at the announced time. During the group sessions, participants may express their common feelings of frustration or joy and share the experiences or insights gained through their hospital work. An experienced member of the volunteer staff may undertake responsibility for leadership functions, contacting interested individuals and facilitating discussion.

Advisory Board

Volunteers (who are more likely to have a long-term, on-going relationship with the child life worker than students) may form an advisory board with the assistance of the child life staff or volunteer services director. The duties of this group might include the organization of programs of special interest to volunteers, advising the child life staff on the needs of volunteers, and assisting in the preparation of future orientation sessions.

Investing Value in the Role of Student and Volunteer

A concern likely to be expressed in meetings such as those described in the preceding section is the feeling of volunteers or students that their roles are insignificant or unnecessary or are held in low esteem by hospital coworkers. While most hospital employees recognize the contribution of these individuals, too often volunteers or students are taken for granted. Volunteers, who work for little more than appreciation and the satisfaction of performing a necessary task, may easily grow dissatisfied if their work becomes unduly repetitious or if its value seems diminished. The child life staff can counteract much of this problem by continually enhancing the volunteer or student's role and imbuing it with a sense of dignity and importance. Among the means of achieving this goal are the following mechanisms:

Schedules

If the volunteer's role is treated by the child life staff as dispensible, it is probable that workers will respond in a like manner. When advising volunteers to "come in when you can," the child life worker communicates the lack of importance attached to the volunteer's position. In effect, volunteers are thus told that their presence is appreciated, but not relied upon. But if volunteers are responsible for a given time period and made aware of the reasons for that assignment, e.g. to provide activities for the many children admitted during evening hours, or to spend morning hours playing with children prior to their surgery, they are likely to develop a sense of commitment to their hospital duties. Furthermore, by assigning volunteers to specific time periods, the child life staff may concentrate their efforts where needed most. When volunteers are unable to work their shift because of illness or another commitment, they should contact the child life supervisor or volunteer director at the earliest possible time. Schedules should also be established for student workers and a similar "call-off" procedure observed.

An added advantage of established hours for volunteers and students, noted by Azarnoff and Flegal (1975), is the opportunity to begin groups of workers at the same time, holding a brief meeting to orient each group to that day's activities. Through these sessions information on children can be transmitted, questions clarified, and particular work assignments made.

Specialized Tasks

Each individual has special talents and interests that they bring to the work assignment. Some prefer work with a specific age-group, while others prefer to concentrate on a particular play medium, e.g., using musical instruments with children or developing creative art projects. Rather than forcing these individuals to fit into a preconceived role of "volunteer" or "student," the child life staff should attempt to build upon the talents of each worker, using their abilities to enhance the total program. The commitment of the volunteers or students to their work will likely increase when given a chance to augment their duties through their valued personal skills.

Communication

Rather than acting as mere overseers of children, students and volunteers are capable of performing an important function by observing the behavior of children and their families. The child life staff can demonstrate the importance of this role to the overall program by establishing clearly defined channels through which these observations may be transmitted. One means of communicating this information is through the previously suggested group meetings at the beginning of each activity period or "shift." At the conclusion of each volunteer or student shift, a brief meeting can be held with the child life supervisor to relate experiences which the workers believe significant. Since some workers may conclude their work period after the child life supervisor has left the hospital, an alternative or supplementary mechanism may be employed. For example, a log may be kept in the child life office in which volunteers or students may briefly record significant observations made during their shift.

Information received by the child life worker through the established channels should be evaluated, with appropriate notations made in the records of the patients observed. In this way, observations of students and volunteers are available to assist other members of the health care team in the planning and evaluation of patient care. It is most desirable if students serving an internship in the child life department do their own charting, under the supervision of the child life staff. In settings where this is not allowed, however, the child life supervisor should record the observations as described.

Continuing Educational Experiences

The value with which students and volunteers are regarded may be further demonstrated through the opportunity to participate in periodic educational experiences. Workers can be informed of meetings, speakers, and inservice sessions occurring in the hospital on topics relevant to their child life duties. In addition, special programs on subjects of importance to volunteers and students can be developed and presented by the child life department and other disciplines. When these opportunities fall during workers' shifts, they should be allowed time off to attend. The provision of educational experiences not only benefits volunteers and students, whose duties are made more interesting and meaningful through increased knowledge, but also benefits child life programming as a whole, which receives the services of more sophisticated personnel.

Evaluation

While formal evaluation is commonly incorporated into the work experiences of students in hospitals, the practice is less frequently used in dealing with volunteers. Child life supervisors may consider scheduling periodic evaluation conferences with volunteers, and also may wish to develop a written progress sheet for use at these intervals. By asking volunteers to participate in evaluation conferences, the child life staff indicates the seriousness with which they view the efforts of these individuals. The evaluation process should not, however, be seen as a means of eliminating less productive workers, for this will only serve to increase the anxiety of all. Rather, the sessions should be used to provide valuable feedback on the performance of volunteers, identifying their strengths as well as weaknesses. (See "Guidelines for Giving Feedback on Performance" later in this chapter.)

Honors and Awards

In addition to the efforts of the child life staff to enhance the role of volunteers and students through the methods described above, these workers should occasionally receive formal recognition of their efforts. Upon completing a specified number of hours, volunteers may be awarded service pins or certificates at a banquet or luncheon held in their honor. Such occasions are usually planned and coordinated by the volunteer services director, but if none exists, the child life department may need to take the initiative in honoring its most dedicated volunteers.

SUPERVISING CHILD LIFE STAFF

As valuable as the services of volunteers and students are to the achievement of child life program goals, they cannot replace the consistency or depth of understanding and experience available through the use of full-time professional child life personnel. High quality child life services require well trained, highly committed individuals. But securing approval for a new position or screening applicants and hiring an excellent worker is not all that it takes to obtain high quality service. Staff members must be supervised with at least as much care as that given to volunteers and students.

Orientation for New Child Life Employees

Like volunteers and students, new employees of the child life department must receive an orientation to their new duties. The content of this training, while similar in many respects to that of volunteers and students, will be modified to fit the needs of the individual. For example, since a thorough knowledge of children is a prerequisite for a child life worker and previous experience in medical settings is highly desirable, it will be less necessary for a supervisor to expose new employees to basic information on the normal development of children and their reactions under stress.

Although new child life employees may be required to attend orientation sessions provided for all entering hospital personnel, formal orientation to the child life department will likely be limited, with greater emphasis on "on-the-job" adjustment to new routines. However, all new child life workers should initially be provided with the following information and experiences:

A REVIEW OF THE JOB DESCRIPTION. The duties of the new employee should be thoroughly clarified to avoid misunderstanding at a later date. The presence of ambiguities in the job description or possible modification of duties in the near future should be discussed at this time.

DEPARTMENTAL EXPECTATIONS. New employees should be familiar with the objectives of the child life program. In addition, any specific expectations of the new worker in achieving these objectives should be clarified. For example, an objective might state that each member of the child life department will present at least one inservice for nursing personnel in the coming year.

A Tour of the Hospital.

Introduction to Key Personnel. If the new employee is to function as a member of the health care team, it is important that he or she be introduced to personnel from other disciplines. The new child life worker may find it advisable to arrange "get acquainted" meetings with some of these individuals.

Explanations of Routines. New child life workers should be aware of the general routines followed by children, the established patterns of child life programming, and the schedule of meetings they will be required to attend.

Explanation of Specific Procedures. Child life personnel should be acquainted with those procedures that may be peculiar to the facility, such as specific methods of charting, tabulating statistics on patient contacts, completing daily report sheets, or requisitioning supplies.

A handbook or manual, similar to that prepared for volunteers and students, detailing information pertinent to the performance of their duties, should be given to new child life employees. Supervisors should also be ready to provide support and advice to employees as they adjust to their new responsibilities. Although newly employed child life workers often have had previous work experience and are familiar with the medical setting (an advantage less frequently shared by volunteers and students) they, too, are subject to doubts and conflicting feelings when entering an unfamiliar environment and a new stage of their careers.

Guidelines for Giving Feedback on Performance

Along with the responsibility for supervising volunteers, students, or staff, the child life worker accepts the obligation to evaluate personnel, praising a job well done, offering suggestions for improved performance, or urging the modification of unacceptable practices. For child life workers unaccustomed to the supervision and management of personnel, the experience of giving feedback on performance to subordinates may be foreign and threatening. One fears that important, yet sensitive, matters will not be properly addressed, resulting either in limited effectiveness in producing change or in the disintegration of relations with the personnel supervised. To facilitate the efforts of child life supervisors when approaching this task, the following guidelines are offered:

Elicit the Subordinate's Assessment. Begin by urging the other person to assess his or her performance or to describe the problem behavior under consideration before *you* describe it.

Listen Attentively. Listen carefully to the subordinate's assessment, without interrupting, even though you may not agree with what the person is saying. Refer to the guidelines for active listening included in Chapter 3.

Describe the Subordinate's Performance. After hearing the person's perception of his or her own performance, describe the performance as you see it. Try to describe the behavior only. Tell how the behavior looks, sounds, and feels to you, without interpreting the behavior or motives of the person. For example, it is better to say, "You focus your attention on only one child in the playroom," than "You seem afraid to get involved with playroom groups."

AVOID THE USE OF EMOTIONALLY CHARGED WORDS. Try to avoid using words such as "hostile," "uncooperative," "disorganized," "domineering," etc., in assessing the performance of others. Instead, describe the *behavior* that led you to infer these characteristics. For example, say "You often speak in a gruff tone and frown," instead of "You're often hostile." Or say "You submit orders for materials only after your current supply has run out," rather than "You're disorganized."

DISCUSS THE CONSEQUENCES OF THE SUBORDINATE'S BEHAVIOR. Instead of moralizing or judging ("It's irresponsible to leave the siderail down on a child's bed!"), point out the natural consequences of the behavior ("If you leave the siderail down on a child's bed, it's likely that he or she may fall").

LIMIT THE FOCUS OF THE DISCUSSION. Do not flood the person with so many different pieces of information that he or she feels overwhelmed. Focus only on a limited number of problem areas.

IGNORE CONDITIONS THE SUBORDINATE CANNOT CONTROL. It is not helpful to focus on conditions over which the person has no control such as a pronounced accent or diminutive size.

OFFER CONCRETE SUGGESTIONS FOR IMPROVEMENT. Be specific about what the person could do to improve. Make specific suggestions for behavior changes, even if you are not sure the person will accept them. For example, say "Position yourself in the playroom so you can view the activities of all children," rather than "Supervise playroom activities more closely." Or, say "Try to make small talk with at least three members of the nursing staff," instead of "Try to be friendlier to the nurses."

EMPHASIZE POSITIVE BEHAVIOR. Find as many behaviors as possible to which you can respond positively. Remember that positive feedback promotes growth at least as efficiently as criticism.

CHECK THE SUBORDINATE'S UNDERSTANDING. As the person to summarize what you have said in order to check how clearly you have communicated. During times of high anxiety, listeners often distort what they have heard. Be prepared to clarify and explain again.

Formulating Objectives with the Child Life Staff

The evaluation of permanent employees is imbued with a special significance, less present in the assessment of students or volunteers. The staff member's continued employment, financial advancement, or assumption of new responsibilities may be dependent upon the supervisor's submission of a favorable progress report. If the criteria for evaluation are ambiguously stated and a satisfactory rating is left to the supervisor's interpretation of these poorly defined categories, the potential for conflict between the supervisor and staff member increases.

For example, a supervisor's rating of a subordinate's level of cooperation as "unsatisfactory" may be viewed as an arbitrary expression of the superior's generalized dissatisfaction with the employee. Such an assessment may easily result in the employee's resentment, damaging the potential for a workable relationship with the supervisor.

The child life supervisor may avoid problems of this nature by meeting with personnel a considerable period of time prior to the evaluation, to agree upon categories for future assessment and to establish objective means of measuring the employee's performance. Thus, rather than labelling a subordinate as "satisfactory" in the area of cooperation, the child life supervisor can make the objective assessment that the employee has achieved the predetermined goals of attending a specified number of meetings, submitting reports on time, and participating in other established functions.

More than merely a means of producing effective employee evaluations, the system of formulating objectives with employees provides for efficient management of the child life department. The objectives established for individual employees may be incorporated into larger departmental objectives, thereby affirming a direction for the department and ploting the means through which these goals will be attained. Although the precise method of formulating child life department goals will vary with the setting, the following steps offer basic guidelines for this process:

Discuss Departmental Goals

A meeting of the child life staff should be convened for a free-ranging discussion of the past performance of the child life department, possible areas for improvement, and new projects to be pursued. The child life supervisor may ask that each member come prepared with a list of potential objectives for the year. It is important to elicit the ideas of all staff members, so that each may feel part of the goals ultimately selected.

The process of establishing departmental goals is too important to be rushed through in a brief staff meeting at the end of a busy day, when people are tired and preoccupied. The staff needs to be away from the interruptions and distractions that are inevitable in the hospital, and they need adequate time to talk through plans and problems thoughtfully. One of the authors has utilized a "Think Day" as a vehicle for setting departmental goals. The staff arrange for volunteers to maintain basic services to patients in their absence and hold a day-long meeting at a location away from the hospital. Without the time pressure that usually characterizes staff meetings, personnel are able to listen thoughtfully to the ideas of others and arrive at goals that represent a genuine consensus.

Define Specific Objectives

From among the many suggestions for possible departmental goals, the staff must agree on those that will be given highest priority during the coming year. These must then be phrased very specifically, describing the type of result desired, rather than using broad, ambiguous labels. For example, rather than saying, "The child life staff will improve its interaction with other disciplines," an objective might state that "A child life representative will attend each of three weekly health care team meetings," or "One member each from the departments of nursing, psychology, and social work will participate in the orientation of new child life volunteers."

The period of time permitted for the achievement of each objective should be determined and specified. Also included are the means of measuring success in attaining the selected goals. The objectives cited above are readily measurable, since attendance at health care team meetings is recorded in the minutes and participation of other disciplines in orientation sessions is easily observable by those present. For other examples of methods of evaluating the successful achievement of objectives, refer to the section on evaluation in Chapter 10.

Set Individual Objectives to Meet Departmental Goals

The successful attainment of departmental goals depends on the efforts of individual department members. Therefore, each department member should undertake the accomplishment of certain objectives designed to facilitate overall goals. For example, each child life worker may agree to attend one health care team meeting per week or to arrange for the participation of one member of another discipline in an up-coming orientation session, in order that the departmental goals are achieved.

Establish Personal Objectives

In consultation with the child life supervisor, individual staff members may have identified specific areas in their performance requiring improvement or continued development. The employee and supervisor should identify the specific behavior changes desired and establish measurable objectives designed to produce the change. For example, the child life worker who seldom reorders materials until existing supplies are exhausted might agree to perform weekly inventories of supplies, submitting a purchase order for items needed every Friday.

Evaluate Performance at Specified Intervals

When the period for the attainment of objectives has lapsed, the child life supervisor should meet again with department members individually and as a group. During individual evaluation sessions the supervisor and staff member review both the individual objectives tied to departmental goals and those objectives for the employee's personal performance. By referring to the specific means of measuring the success in achieving each goal, the supervisor and staff member can readily determine the progress made by the individual, without relying on the caprices of subjective opinions.

Following individual sessions, the staff should meet as a group to assess the progress of the department and to reevaluate its direction. With this meeting, the process of formulating new objectives for the child life department begins once again.

The management of a department through the continual formulation of measurable objectives offers the child life supervisor several important advantages. First, it provides a sense of direction for departmental efforts, avoiding unnecessary stagnation or the random discharge of unchanneled energy. Second, the process provides for the objective determination of the success of child life programming, documentation of which will be invaluable when seeking continued or increased support from the hospital. Finally, and perhaps most importantly, the process demands the active involvement of all personnel, increasing their communication with other staff members and clearly linking their individual efforts to the success of the total program.

CHAPTER 10

"SELLING" A CHILD LIFE PROGRAM

THE FUTURE OF CHILD LIFE

B oth Rita and Roberta are being rushed to the hospital with suspected meningitis. Both are four years old. Both have no idea of what a hospital is like. Both leave confused, upset siblings behind them at home. Both have parents who are worried and frightened. Both will receive the medical care necessary to save them from this serious illness.

But there the similarity ends. Rita will adjust readily to the hospital stay and will return home chattering to her friends about her latest experience. Roberta will cry herself to sleep every night in the hospital and will remain withdrawn and cling to her mother for weeks after she returns home.

What accounts for the difference between the two stories? Rita was lucky enough to live near a children's hospital with a well-established child life program. Roberta, through no fault of her own, lives in a small city and will be admitted to one of the many general hospitals with no child life services.

For any other child in the United States or Canada, the likelihood of having an experience like Rita's is still slim, since fewer than one percent of the hospitals admitting children have established child life programs. The overwhelming majority of children in North America face the prospect of hospitalization without the support and understanding that will help Rita return home as well emotionally as she will be medically.

Although the preceding chapters, with their glowing accounts of what child life services can offer children and their parents, may give the impression that child life is a well-established discipline, in reality it is a field with a brief history but a promising future.

In his survey of child life programs in the United States, Rutkowski (1978) discovered that the average age of a program was only 11.35 years. Mather and Glasrud (1980) found a similar figure: 12 years. In interpreting Rutkowski's data, Larsen (1980) pointed out that

up to 1949, the end of the first decade [of the existence of child life programs], only 10% of the 120 programs studied were in existence. During the 1950's another 13% were established. The most phenomenal growth has taken place between 1960 and 1976 [the date of Rutkowski's survey], when 77% of the 120 programs were founded. . . . Rutkowski discovered that the peak period of growth was during the three-year period of 1968 to 1970, when 25% of all 120 programs were founded. . . . Despite this noteworthy peak, the overall rate of growth during the 1970's was still considerably higher than that of the 1960's (p. 3).

In addition to new programs being established, existing programs have been expanding in recent years. Rutkowski notes that 87 percent of the surveyed programs had experienced growth since their inception. Larsen also notes that the staff of the program she heads (Montreal Children's Hospital) has doubled in the past decade and suggests that this "is probably not an uncommon experience (p. 3)."

When one considers that approximately 3000 hospitals in the U.S. and Canada serve children and that the most recent edition of the *Directory of Child Life Activity Programs in North America* (ACCH, 1979) lists only some 270 hospitals with child life programs, the need for continued expansion is obvious. Many hundreds of hospitals are "candidates" for child life programming, even if they have not yet decided to institute a program.

In a survey conducted in 1978 (Stanford, 1979), 207 (or 45%) of the responding hospitals indicated that they "do" or "perhaps" foresee hiring one or more child life workers within the next five years. Perhaps even more significantly, fully 55 of the responding hospitals indicated that they would like to be contacted by a qualified person to discuss the possibility of developing a child life program at their hospital.

Not only is it reasonable to anticipate continued expansion in the number and size of child life programs, but it is also possible to predict the nature of the hospitals that are likely to institute new child life programs. Since almost every major children's hospital already has a child life program and since children's hospitals represent only about 2 percent of the medical facilities that serve children, it can be assumed that the future of child life lies in smaller, community hospitals rather than in specialized facilities for children. That is, the programs that are established in the coming years are almost certain to be in general hospitals with pediatric units of, say, 15 to 40 beds.

The establishment of a new child life program in this type of hospital will come about in one of two ways: Either the impetus will come from within the institution, with existing hospital personnel realizing the need for child life programming and creating one or more new positions for which trained professionals will be recruited; or it will come from outside the institution, with someone, such as a parent or a recently trained Child Life Specialist, convincing the hospital that a child life program would improve their service to children.

Both approaches to new programming will require considerable "selling." In the first situation, the "selling" of the child life program will come chiefly *after* the new child life worker is hired. In the latter, it must take place *before* a new position is created. Techniques for accomplishing both types of "selling" are the focus of the present chapter, which will begin, most logically, with a review of the hospital conditions that give rise to the need for child life programming.

WHEN CHILD LIFE IS ABSENT

The research of more than 30 years has consistently demonstrated the importance of providing children with specialized forms of support when facing the stressful event of hospitalization. Children need the presence and support of their parents, not merely for limited periods of visitation, but as an integral component of their care. For parents to fulfill this function, while themselves under stress, the hospital must provide for their physical and emotional needs. Hospitalized children and their families need explanations of unaccustomed procedures, equipment, and events, presented in a sensitive, comprehensible manner, to reduce the unfamiliarity of the medical environment. Children in hospitals also need play experiences, to promote their normal development during the period away from home, and to minimize the potential for psychological trauma. Through the provision of these services and opportunities, children and their parents develop relationships of trust with members of the hospital staff, which help sustain them through the periods of most severe stress.

Child life programs have developed as a means of insuring that services essential to the emotional well-being of hospitalized children and their families are readily available. Personnel in those facilities lacking effective child life programs are likely to encounter problems in the care and management of children. For example, those children who have limited play experiences are liable to be more depressed and less well-adjusted than children able to attain a feeling of mastery through the active manipulation of play materials. When hostile feelings are encouraged to find expression through play experiences, they are less likely to appear in more harmful forms, such as violence towards others, sleep disturbances, nightmares, or other lingering manifestations of psychological upset.

Similarly, a failure to understand the meaning or purpose of a new experience may cause anxiety in children and parents which frustrates the patient's treatment. A child who has been adequately prepared for the induction of anesthesia and is cognizant of its benefits, as well as anticipated unpleasantness such as a funny smell or the prick of a needle, will likely face the event with a greater sense of calm and control than the child who must rely on inner fantasies as a source of explanations. The unprepared child may well face the horror of being restrained by masked strangers while unconsciousness is induced.

Hospitals may permit parents to room in and visit their children 24 hours a day, but, unless someone is responsible for managing parent services, monitoring their concerns and mediating conflicts that may arise due to their presence, chaos may result. Staff members who feel that their ability to care for children satisfactorily is hampered by parental presence may, through their open resentment and hostility, discourage the participation of parents. Parents, on the other hand, who lack guidance and a clear understanding of their role in the medical setting may be incapable of providing support to their children, despite the staff's tolerance of their presence. In either case, the effectiveness of a parenting program is greatly diminished.

IMPETUS FOR CHILD LIFE FROM WITHIN

Problems of these types will lead hospital personnel, in some cases, to take the initiative in correcting those concerns by pursuing the establishment of child life programming. A position is therefore created and a professional recruited who is given a mandate to develop those services viewed by hospital personnel as essential to the solution of their problems.

Since most major hospitals dealing in the care of children already have some form of child life programming, the type of hospital likely to seek a professional to establish a new child life program is a smaller community or general hospital. The total number of pediatric beds in such facilities, though varying from a few to as many as 50 beds, will typically be fewer than in a major institution. Due to the smaller bed capacity, it is probable that the child life worker, at least initially, will work without assistance. In such facilities, the pediatric unit is only one of a number of areas, serving the entire life span and broad range of conditions.

These characteristics of the community or general hospital, i.e. smaller pediatric unit and broader service orientation, will affect the structure of the child life programming developed. Of principal importance is the fact that departments such as admitting, X-ray, laboratory, dietary, and many others serve patients of all ages, and therefore the personnel in each may be less inclined to become experts in the care of children. The laboratory technician who draws blood from children in the pediatric unit may next travel to the coronary care unit and then to the maternity ward. Amid such a schedule it is difficult for the technician to acquire a keen awareness of the needs of children of various ages and to modify techniques accordingly.

Similarly, the attention of other support groups, generally available in major children's facilities to coordinate with and supplement services to child life programming, is divided among several patient areas. Social work, for example, may be less able to provide assistance in the coordination of services for parents; or volunteer services, concerned with providing help to all hospital areas, may be prevented from participating in a pediatric preadmission orientation program.

The relatively minor position of the pediatric unit in the total hospital structure may also have great influence on the environment to which children are subjected. According to Dr. Edward R. Duffie, Jr.:

> In most general hospitals, the pediatric census runs between five and 10 percent of the total patient load, though in a few very active pediatric wards of general hospitals, it may run as much as 15 to 20 percent. As a result, the pediatric service generally comes out second best in the competition for dollars, personnel, space, and equipment, especially when competing with strong internal medicine, surgery, laboratory, and other departments (Oremland & Oremland, 1973, p. 299).

Because of the weaker position of pediatrics, it is less likely that a general hospital will readily pursue the adaptation of the environment of areas such as admitting, X-ray department, laboratory, and surgical waiting areas for the benefit of children.

The child life worker hired to establish child life programming in a general hospital setting under circumstances such as those described faces a monumental task. In addition to the establishment of a play program for the children, the individual will undoubtedly see the need for a variety of other services. Personnel, such as admitting clerks, X-ray technicians, and laboratory workers, who have limited contact with children may need to receive inservice training on the reactions of children to hospitalization and effective techniques for communicating with children and parents. The child life worker may wish to expand the services presently provided for parents or institute preadmission tours and surgical preparation. Finally, the child life worker may see an acute need to serve as an advocate for pediatric patients, seeking changes that will promote more sensitive care throughout the institution.

Simultaneous development of all desired services is, of course, impossible, but as the more immediate and essential elements of programming are successfully established, the child life worker may begin work on other goals. The pediatric census is characteristically mercurial. During periods of low patient occupancy the child life worker can concentrate more fully on additional projects of highest priority.

The child life worker may find, however, that problems with other staff members arise as attention is turned from initial goals to the institution of other services. As mentioned earlier, when individuals within an organization identify problems in the care of children and seek the establishment of child life programming to solve those problems, the child life worker hired for the position is given a mandate to perform certain functions. Should he or she then attempt to expand from the primary program for which he or she was hired to begin offering other services essential to the care of children in general hospitals, resistance may be felt.

For example, the pediatric nursing staff in a general hospital in a small city in the Midwest recognized the value of play in helping children express their feelings about hospitalization and gain mastery in a powerless situation. Accordingly, they, with the assistance of the hospital administrator, recruited a child life worker to establish a therapeutic play program. After a short period in the hospital, it became apparent to the child life worker that much of the distress children expressed through their play was caused by their lack of knowledge about the environment and procedures. Therefore, the child life worker attempted to institute a preparation program with the assistance of Nursing. Having had so much cooperation and success with the play program, she was puzzled by Nursing's rather cool reception to her ideas for a preparation program. To gain their support required several times more effort than it did to get the play program off the ground.

The principles for coping with resistance to child life programming discussed in Chapter 8 may be applied by individuals hired to establish programs in community or general hospitals when attempting to expand the focus of their work. Sources of potential resistance among personnel should be anticipated and analyzed, with appropriate interventions employed to counter its effects.

For example, the child life worker who considered the introduction of a preparation program important for the general hospital pediatric patients might inform others of its value through various means such as inservice presentations and the dissemination of articles. The competent presentation of this information and the efforts to involve other personnel in the process would reassure those who might be reluctant to support the program. Ultimately, the individuals who sought the original programming (in this case, the nursing staff who wanted the play program) will find that the expansion of child life services in this way conforms to the overall goal of reducing the emotional upset of children. Further mechanisms for increasing the support for child life programming, both within and outside the hospital, will be discussed later in the present chapter.

"CREATING" A JOB IN CHILD LIFE

In the preceding section disussion focused on the situation in which hospital personnel, aware of problems in the care of children that could be solved by instituting a child life program, took the initiative to begin a program and sought a trained individual to help them achieve their goal. In other situations that lack child life programs, hospital personnel may either fail to see the conditions in the hospital that are creating emotional upset in children or may lack the initiative to implement change by starting a child life program. In these instances, staff members may feel a generalized discontent about the situation, but they accept the unpleasant element as an inevitable part of the performance of their duties. For example, the nursing staff may accept depression among hospitalized children as distressing, but unalterable, or may view the destructive, hostile behavior of children as an inevitable side-effect of hospitalization. Operating room personnel may detest their role in restraining obviously frightened children, yet may see no alternative to this unpleasant task. When the initiative for instituting solutions to commonly held problems through child life programming does not arise from within the hositai, the impetus must come from concerned individuals outside the organization.

The traditional job-finding methods of scouring classified pages for available positions and widely disseminating copies of one's resumé will be of little help to the professional seeking a child life position in these hospitals. Although the need for child life services exists, individuals within the organization are not yet familiar with the value to be gained from child life. A more deliberate approach must be formulated if hospital personnel are to become aware of the benefits of child life programming and then seek implementation of its services in solving their problems.

An alternative approach, well-suited to the task of introducing child life programming to new hospital settings or creating new jobs in those programs that already exist, is offered by Richard N. Bolles (1978). His method of job-searching, designed to help the general job-hunter in pursuit of a satisfying position, basically consists of the following steps:

(1) Decide exactly what you want to do.

(2) Decide exactly where you want to do it.

(3) Thoroughly research the organizations that interest you to find:
    (a) who within the organization is in a position to hire you, and
    (b) what problems that person has that you can solve with the skills you possess.

Although a time-consuming process, this method of locating a position suited to the skills of the individual allows the job-seeker more control and certainly promises more success than the less directed, traditional approaches, such as waiting for a child life job to be advertised in the want-ads. The applicability of Bolles' method to child life workers, particularly those wishing to establish new programs, will be explored below.

Decide Exactly What You Want To Do

For those interested in child life work, the basic perimeter of this decision is already established: a career in a program providing emotional support to hospitalized children and their families is sought. Yet, after drawing these boundaries, a number of considerations remain. For example, one must decide whether to seek a position in a preexisting program to establish a new one. What exact form of child life work is desired? The job-seeker must decide whether to pursue an in-patient position or one in an out-patient clinic or emergency room. If in an inpatient setting, does the individual wish to work with a broad range of children or prefer specializing in children of a certain age or medical condition, e.g. children with spinal cord injuries, emotional problems, or a particular disease such as cancer.

Decide Exactly Where You Want to Work

In deciding exactly where to work, the individual is actually making two basic choices, each of which are dependent on other phases of the job search. First, the child life worker must select a geographic location, based on his or her personal tastes. Practical considerations must, however, enter into this selection process. After deciding the nature of the job one wishes to do and determining the desired location, thorough research of the organization must ensue. A child life worker living on the east coast, wanting to work in San Francisco will have a difficult time conducting research on hospitals in this distant location, unless the commitment is made to move to the desired area for an extended period. Thus, when deciding on a geographic location, child life workers must choose an area that is accessible for investigation from their present location.

A further practical consideration in selecting the desired geographic location is whether the area is likely to offer a "fertile field" for job hunting. Particularly, one must assess the popularity of a given area among other professionals, and weigh this popularity against an estimate of the number of child life jobs the area is likely to support. For example, a highly popular, "vacation-type" setting such as Provincetown, Massachusetts, may have a relatively low number of permanent residents and a single hospital with a small pediatric unit already served by a child life worker. Chances of successfully obtaining a satisfactory position in this area will be low, and therefore the individual must exercise some flexibility in the desired location.

A survey conducted by Stanford (1979) offers the only data on possible job opportunities in child life broken down by geographic area. The survey was taken in the summer of 1978, by mailing questionnaires to all hospital-based pediatricians in the United States, all English-speaking pediatricians in Canada, personnel directors of all U.S. hospitals with more than 100 beds and all children's hospitals regardless of size, the personnel directors of all Canadian hospitals, and all directors of child life programs listed in the ACCH *Directory.*

The responding hospitals that indicated that they either "do" or "perhaps" foresee hiring one or more child life workers within the next five years were examined to determine into what geographic region most of them fall. On the following page is a rank ordering of the regions, from greatest percentage of positive responses to lowest percentage of positive responses.

Percentages do not tell the entire story, however. When only absolute numbers are considered, the greatest number of positive responses came from the Northeastern United States, followed by (in descending order)

Percentage of responding hospitals that might hire a child life worker	Region
59%	Canada
49%	South Central United States (Texas, Missouri, Louisiana, Oklahoma, Arkansas, Mississippi)
47%	Southeastern United States (Tennessee, South Carolina, North Carolina, Kentucky, Georgia, Alabama, Maryland, West Virginia, Florida, Virginia)
45%	Southwestern United States (California, Arizona, Colorado, New Mexico, Utah, Nevada)
42%	Northeastern United States (Rhode Island, Ohio, New York, New Jersey, Indiana, New Hampshire, Michigan, Massachusetts, Delaware, Pennsylvania, Connecticut, Maine, Vermont)
40%	Northwestern United States (Oregon, Washington Montana, Idaho, Alaska, Hawaii, Wyoming)
35%	North Central United States (Wisconsin, North Dakota, Iowa, Minnesota, South Dakota, Illinois, Nebraska, Kansas)

Southeastern United States, Canada, South Central United States, North Central United States, Southwestern United States, Northwestern United States. In other words, although there may be greater *relative* interest in hiring child life workers in some other parts of the country and Canada, the most potential jobs lie in the Northeast, probably because there are simply more hospitals in that region because it contains the big population centers.

Aside from deciding upon a given geographic area, child life workers must also select the individual institutions in which they wish to work. The selection of these facilities will be influenced by the decision made concerning the exact nature of the work desired. For example, if an individual wishes to establish a new child life program, hospitals within the chosen geographic area presently lacking such programming, yet serving pediatric patients, must be identified. On the other hand, if a particular speciality is desired, such as working with oncology patients, the child life worker will likely have to look to a larger facility with a currently existing child life program.

Other factors may be considered in the selection of a particular facility. The child life worker may be attracted to the philosophy of patient care of a given hospital or to the potential for improving the physical setting. The receptivity of the staff members to change, the size of the hospital or pediatric unit, or the degree of community support for the facility are among other elements that may influence an individual to pursue a position in a particular hospital within the favored geographic location.

Thoroughly Research the Selected Organizations

The majority of the child life worker's time spent in the job-hunting process will likely be devoted to the thorough investigation of the organization or organizations selected through the preceding process. The goal of this exhaustive research is to discover (1) who within the institution has the power to hire you, and (2) what problems that individual may have that you can eliminate with the skills in your possession.

Sources of Information

The imaginative researcher will discover a wealth of information available on the institution in question. Much of this information will be derived from direct contact with the facility and its employees. Public relations materials and informational pamphlets produced by the hospital will be of some help in identifying its philosophical stance, administrative officers, and programs presently in existence, but will do little to uncover problems existing within the institution.

For that information the prospective child life worker may turn to personal interviews with members of the hospital staff. Although an understanding of the concerns of staff associated with pediatric patients is an ultimate goal of the interviewing process, these discussions may begin with most any hospital employee. Through this individual, perhaps a friend or acquaintance of the job-seeker, other members of the hospital staff may be introduced. In the absence of an initial contact person in the hospital, the child life worker may, instead, directly contact hospital personnel such as the head nurse of pediatrics, the director of social services, or an assistant administrator, using mutual interest in the health care of children as a basis of discussion.

Another portion of the research may be conducted outside of the hospital. Local newspapers may, for example, be a source of pertinent information. As with the printed matter procured in the hospital, newspaper articles appearing through the efforts of the facility's public relations department will reflect a basic view toward patient care. Of greater help in the job search, however, will be those articles about the hospital or local health care generated from sources other than representatives of the institution. For example, an article revealing the decline of occupancy rates in the hospital's pediatric unit or a letter to the editor either praising or criticizing the care of children in the facility can be helpful in forming a picture of hospital needs.

Parents whose children have recently been hospitalized in the institution being researched are an invaluable source of information. Their perceptions are most helpful in identifying problems, such as low morale among pediatric nurses or difficulty in managing the behavior of patients, as well as positive aspects, such as the staff's desire to implement a preparation program or up-grade the environment. In addition to contacting individual parents, the researcher should be in communication with local parents organizations, exploring their understanding of the needs and assets of local pediatric care.

The prospective child life worker may further contact personnel employed by other hospitals in the area. The child life worker or members of the pediatric staff of Hospital *X* may have valuable insights into the situation at Hospital *Y*, offering reasons for the lack of child life programming to date and identifying probable sources of resistance or support in the present attempts to institute such services.

Who Is in a Position to Hire You?

Through the exhaustive research process, the investigator will have developed an understanding of the hospital organization and will have identified the individual or individuals within the institution capable of creating a child life position. In many cases, the hospital administrator will be that individual. Even when the impetus for a new position comes from a source other than the administrator, that official is still likely to be involved in the process, requiring a written program proposal for approval of the board of trustees, for example.

The ability to create a new position is not, however, the exclusive province of the hospital administrator. An investigation of power relationships within the institution may reveal that the board of trustees frequently assumes a very active role in initiating policy, which the administrator then executes. Under such conditions it may be more advisable to view the Chairman of the Board as the potential employer. Similarly, a physician such as the chief of staff or chief of pediatrics may be an individual who asserts sufficient authority to create a child life position.

At times, the directors of various departments will be granted permission to expand their departments by a specified number of positions in a given time period. Within those limitations, the director may be free to allocate those positions as desired. Thus, it may be within the power of a director of nursing to forego the hiring of an additional staff nurse in favor of a child life worker. Although the heads of departments such as social services, mental health, or nursing may not have the authority to create new positions at will, circumstances may be such that they are the prospective child life worker's strongest ally in the securing of a job. During the research period the child life worker should carefully consider the role of these individuals, weighing their ability to help obtain that position, their support of child life programming, and the merits of having their departments be a home for child life.

Problems of the Prospective Employer

The next step in the job-search is finding a satisfactory answer to the question, "What problems does the prospective employer have that I can solve with the skills I possess?" Even the most casual investigation of a complex organization such as a hospital is likely to uncover the existence of a number of problems of varying severity. An exhaustive search will yield more than can be meaningfully used. Thus, it is necessary to have some guidelines for determining the relevance of each to the job-search process. Bolles (1978) offers the following suggestions for selecting those problems that will be of value in convincing a prospective employer to create a new position:

THERE IS NO NEED TO DISCOVER ALL PROBLEMS OF THE ORGANIZATION. Only those actually pertaining to the person in a position to hire you are relevant to the job-search process. If, for example, it has been determined that the hospital administrator is the individual who can create a new position, problems that are more likely the concern of the director of nursing, such as the inability of nurses to cope with certain patients, will be of less importance. These problems will, however, be important in shaping the child life program once instituted.

THE PROBLEMS NEED NOT BE HUGE. The problems of the prospective employer may, from your perspective, be relatively minor, yet will be valuable in establishing child life programming if they can be solved with the skills you possess. The director of nursing's concern that the playroom is seldom used may, for example, be easily remedied by simple rearrangement of the area and by the provision of attractive activities.

TRY TO "READ THE MIND" OF THE PROSPECTIVE EMPLOYER. Bolles notes that the prospective employer may be unaware of many of the problems discovered during the research process, although within that individual's authority. Such problems will be of less value in moving the prospective employer to create a new position than those of which the person is already aware and troubled. Thus, Bolles suggests "reading the mind" of the employer, or identifying those problems that are already of concern to the individual, rather than attempting to "educate" the person about new ones.

In the process of identifying problems in a hospital that currently has no child life programming, the prospective child life worker enjoys a considerable advantage. A number of problems, such as those discussed at the beginning of the chapter, will doubtlessly exist due to the very absence of services such as organized therapeutic and developmental play experiences, preparation, and parent support services. The potential for devastating trauma to the child and family is greatly reduced through such programming. Children can express their frustrations and anxieties through their play rather than inappropriate means that endanger their own well-being and aggravate the staff. Parents who receive increased information and support from special services grow less anxious and are better able to offer support to their children. Settings that fail to provide such services will likely produce more depressed or hostile children and a higher degree of anxiety among parents. This condition may lead to strained relationships between staff and parents, or may decrease the level of employee morale.

Knowing the benefits of child life programming to children and their families and the hazards of its absence, the prospective child life worker must reinterpret these strengths to meet the needs of the employer. For example, a paramount goal of child life programming is to reduce the potential for post-hospital upset in children; yet this strength, while desirable, may not be as persuasive to a hospital administrator who is more concerned about the rapid decline in pediatric bed occupancy. Thus, while not sacrificing the goals of such programs, the child life worker may instead emphasize the satisfaction among children and parents that generally results from the introduction of these services. Increased satisfaction among users of the facility is likely to lead to greater utilization by the community as a whole. Likewise, an administrator concerned about the hospital's public image or seeking increased sources of community financial support will be alert to the public relations potential of improved pediatric services.

Similar reinterpretations can be made for prospective employers from other disciplines. For example, the chief of staff, alert to difficulties experienced by anesthesiologists with pediatric patients, may be impressed by the potential of preoperative preparation for reducing this problem. A director of nursing might similarly be impressed by the use of preparation and therapeutic play in reducing the fears of children that often provoke resistance to nursing procedures. The possibility of increased communication with parents and monitoring of their concerns through child life programming may be viewed by the director of social services as an important asset in minimizing the frequent discontent of parents. Through the reinterpretation of benefits of child life programming, the prospective employer gains a sense of the immediate impact the institution of such services can have on the elimination of troublesome problems.

The Interview

Having established the identity of the prospective employer and discovered some problems faced by that person (reinterpreting the goals of child life programming to demonstrate their influence on the solution of the problems), the child life worker must personally contact the individual. Bolles (1978) observes that the formal job interview is often a stressful situation for both parties involved. The prospective employee is under the spotlight and must make an attractive presentation, or the possibility of employment is lost. The employer, on the other hand, feels compelled to make a decision whether to hire or not in a relatively brief period. As an alternative, the child life worker should attempt to create a low stress situation through which the prospective employer has a chance to meet and interact with the job-seeker, without having to make an immediate decision.

The child life worker may be referred to the prospective employer by another person within the organization who was met during the course of the research. The prospective employer may, indeed, have been contacted previously during the investigation. If no such contact has been made, the child life worker may try another approach. The child life worker may consider writing an article on health care and children and wish to interview the prospective employer in this regard. If a student, the child life worker may meet with the employer in conjunction with classwork. The individual may also be contacted to discuss interests, mutually held with the child life worker, in the field of pediatric health care.

Whatever the pretext for scheduling the meeting, the contact allows the prospective employer to, in Bolles' term, "windowshop" the child life worker, evaluating the talents of this individual. With no pressure to make an immediate decision, the employer may conduct a relaxed discussion of his or her role in hospital affairs and the challenges currently confronting that position. During the meeting, the child life worker should be careful to allow the prospective employer to present his or her perception of problem situations before suggesting previously considered solutions. By so doing, the child life worker avoids the mistake of proposing solutions to problems about which the employer is no longer concerned.

For example, the administrator, once concerned about the hospital's public image, may be satisfied with progress made through the production of hospital-sponsored, health-related public service announcements. The child life worker who fails to wait for the administrator's articulation of the problem may prematurely blurt out a solution that indicates to the administrator that this individual has little new or valuable to offer.

If the child life worker's research has been thorough and accurate in identifying the person with the ability to create a new position and some problems of concern to that individual, the interview may lead to an offer of a job. Alternatively, this conference may represent the first of a series of meetings designed to explore the establishment of child life programming. If, however, the initial meeting results in a job offer, the child life worker should be prepared to discuss important particulars such as salary, budget, and space requirements (see Chapter 5). One means of organizing this information is through the presentation of a formal program proposal.

PREPARATION OF A FORMAL PROGRAM PROPOSAL

When negotiating for the establishment of child life services or attempting to expand the scope of an already-existing program, the child life worker may be asked to present a formal proposal or may independently develop one. An instrument of this sort can be a valuable mechanism for effectively arguing the merits of a proposed change, if properly prepared. In addition to describing the nature of the new or expanded programming, a formal proposal can educate the official reviewing it, explaining the genesis of child life programming in other settings and its proven value. Practical matters such as sources of funding, space requirements, and means of evaluating the effectiveness of the proposed change are directly addressed by this document. The precise format of the proposal may vary, possibly being established by institutional policy, but should cover the elements contained in the following outline:*

   I. Program description (present program—or in the case of a new child life program, the proposed program)
      A. Program objectives
      B. Activities to achieve the program objectives
      C. Evaluation of current status
         1. Strengths
         2. Weaknesses
      D. Historical background
      E. Consequences of curtailing or eliminating the program

  II. Proposed change (omitted for new program proposal)

 III. Budget
      A. Costs
      B. Space requirements
      C. Source of funding

 IV. Method of evaluation

The contents of each section of the outline will be described in detail in the paragraphs that follow:

Program Description

In the case of preexisting child life programs (which one is proposing an expansion of or addition to), a thorough description of present services must be included in the proposal. This information allows the administrator, board member, or other interested party to become more familiar with the department's operation, including its current aspirations and the impediments to their achievement. Through this section the reviewer, who may previously have held a limited or distorted view of child life services, may gain a more comprehensive understanding of the program and, one hopes, will be more convinced of its value. The arguments presented to the reviewer in this section may be used, in turn, by that person to defend the merits of child life in other quarters.

If the proposal presented is for a new child life program, its elements should be modified accordingly. A listing should be made of the *proposed*

---

*Based on a concept suggested by Randall L. O'Donnell, presently administrator of Arkansas Children's Hospital, Little Rock, Arkansas.

objectives and programming, accompanied by a presentation of the current conditions within the hospital that make the institution of these services an urgent necessity.

Program Objectives

Both broad and specific goals of child life programming should be stated under program objectives. Global objectives, such as maximizing the child's continued normal development during hospitalization, are helpful in defining the general mission of child life services. These objectives, however, should be subdivided into more specific objectives which describe the territory defined by the broader goals. Thus, a proposal might include the more specific objectives of increasing the amount of contact between patients by X percent (thus enhancing social development) or decreasing the amount of time children spend in bed by X percent (thus fostering normal physical development).

Activities to Achieve the Program Objectives

The activities presented in this section should directly relate to the objectives stated in the preceding section. For example, to attain the goals of increasing social interaction and normal physical activity, the child life program provides structured play and recreation opportunities for all ages, as well as special events, fieldtrips in and out of the hospital, and informal gatherings. A thorough, specific listing of these activities should be displayed to demonstrate present efforts to meet objectives.

Evaluation of Current Status

Through this section child life workers may present their perception of the present situation, evaluating the progress made toward the stated objectives. The successes of child life programming, such as the establishment of a preparation program or the popular acceptance of new playroom activities, should be emphasized. This demonstrates the competence of the staff and its ability to produce change, characteristics that bode well in the allocation of additional resources. If quantifiable measurements of success exist, such as figures on the increased use of the playroom or decreased time spent by patients in their rooms, they should be included in this section.

Weaknesses in current programming should also be presented, along with a consideration of those factors inhibiting greater progress. If, for example, a goal of increasing participation in preadmission tours has not been met due to the lack of funds to publicize the program or because of inadequate staff to conduct weekend tours, these elements must be disclosed.

Historical Background

Many hospital officials have little understanding of the origin of child life programming either within the hospital or in other institutions. An historical background section permits child life workers to correct this matter by explaining the factors that led to the developing of these services. It is frequently helpful to remind officials of the conditions existing in hospitals prior to the institution of child life programming. Those who have become accustomed to the sight of active, alert children and a compassionate environment may need to recall the sterile silence of pediatric wards in past years to appreciate the advances already made.

The historical background section may also be used as a vehicle for informing officials of the types of child life programming existing in other facilities. If, for example, the purpose for writing a proposal is to establish a preadmission tour program, it will be helpful to include information on successful programming of this sort elsewhere. This information will be particularly persuasive if it indicates that a majority of other similar institutions in the area presently provide this service. Therefore, it is advantageous to research the available programming at neighboring hospitals.

Consequences of Curtailing the Program

What would happen if the present child life program were curtailed or eliminated? A comprehensive review of the detrimental effects of such actions should be presented as a portion of the program proposal to emphasize the essential nature of child life programming, dispelling the idea that the services offered are expendable.

Description of Proposed Changes

Based on the information contained in the preceding portion of the document, proposals for changed or additional programming are presented. If program objectives were not met due to inhibiting deficiencies, then a proposal for additional personnel, funding or space will be developed. If, however, the global goals of child life programming were not achieved due to the absence of needed services, or if new problems encountered reveal a need for the expansion of those goals, then a proposal must be made for new elements of the child life program.

For example, the initial objectives of a child life program may focus on the needs of children for play and preparation, but avoid intervention with parents. A review of services makes it apparent, however, that failure to provide more service for parents has a profound negative effect on children. Therefore, the child life department submits a proposal for additional staff and funding to meet the new objectives of providing information and support to parents. (In proposals for·the establishment of a new child life program, this section will be omitted since the essential information was incorporated in the preceding section.)

Proposed New Objectives

The new objectives of child life programming are stated briefly and specifically. For example, a new goal may be to increase the number of parents of preschoolers who "room-in" with their children or to reduce the anxiety observable in parents.

Activities to Achieve the New Objectives

What type of programming is needed to achieve the newly defined goals? To increase parental participation, it may be necessary to provide improved facilities such as cots, showers and a lounge. The hiring of an additional child life worker may be necessary to coordinate the affairs of parents, to hold daily parents' meetings, and to provide the increased amount of information to parents that can be effective in reducing their anxiety. Activities considered necessary to attain the new goals should be fully delineated.

Reasons for the Proposed Change

In preparing this section of the proposal, the child life staff should carefully describe the conditions indicating a need for change and identify those individuals or groups that seek the new policy. For example, the condition prompting change may be an increasing number of conflicts between parents and the nursing staff, largely due to the inadequacy of facilities provided for parents. The nursing staff, tired of attempting to care for children in cramped quarters, may have requested the proposed changes. The verbal comment of parents or their written hospital evaluations may have indicated the need for improved facilities. Or perhaps a new governmental regulation or recommendation from the Joint Commission for Accreditation of Hospitals mandates the change. Whatever the reasons for pursuing change may be, they should be fully explained and documented.

Budget

Most major changes cannot be accomplished without the allocation of additional personnel, funding, or space. A realistic statement of the resources needed to implement the proposed change (or to start a new child life program) is essential. If a portion of the funding for the project can be obtained from sources other than the hospital budget, include this amount, the name of the organization supplying it, and the balance needed from hospital funds.

As stated in Chapter 5, it is not usually desirable to have the principal source of financial support for child life come from external, temporary sources. Such an arrangement may leave the existence of the child life program vulnerable to the caprices of the funding source. The lack of direct funding from the hospital budget also may indicate an insufficient commitment by the institution to the goals of child life programming. Temporary funding may prove helpful, however, in establishing a child life program when the hospital initially refuses to commit its support. Once hospital personnel become the beneficiaries of child life programming, they will likely be reluctant to lose it. Even so, when arranging for external funding for a pilot child life program, the child life worker should seek the hospital's commitment that demonstration of the program's success will lead to its inclusion in the hospital budget.

Evaluation

The final portion of the proposal is devoted to the important question of evaluation. As concern over the rising cost of health care increases, so will the close scrutiny of hospital spending. For this reason it is insufficient merely to propose programming what *appears* to be of value to hospital personnel and clientele; it is essential to include in the program proposal a method of actually measuring the achievement of the stated objectives. If the hospital is to designate funds for a particular purpose, it wants to insure that its money is well spent. Thus, the child life worker seeking the establishment of a program by the hospital, its continued support, or the expansion of child life services must be able to demonstrate accountability.

A variety of methods exist for evaluating the success of child life programming. The method chosen in each case will depend on the nature of the objective to be measured and on the resources devoted to the process. For example, a simple compilation of statistics is sufficient to measure the objective of increasing family participation in preadmission tours, while a more complex mechanism is needed to measure the effects of child life programming on reducing the psychological upset of children. For the latter, a post-hospital rating scale to be completed by parents may be necessary, or a record kept of the child's vital physiological signs during stressful periods of hospitalization. A review of some of the principal forms of evaluating child life progress follows:

Anecdotal Reports

Anecdotal reports are among the most easily gathered evaluatory data, although least rigorous from a scientific perspective. The child life worker can compile positive comments received from staff, parents, and children concerning the particular service being considered. A tape recorder is a good means of recording these comments, saving the child life worker or the speaker the time and effort of putting thoughts on paper. While not easily quantifiable, the words of an appreciative parent or child can be highly persuasive in the decision to continue or expand a certain program.

Written Evaluation Forms

Questionnaires or checklists, designed to measure the value or effectiveness of selected aspects of child life programming as perceived by parents or children, may be produced by the child life staff, perhaps in consultation with other hospital personnel. Statistics derived from these evaluation forms may be used to measure the success of the new program, while solicitation of additional comments helps the staff modify the program to better meet the needs of the individuals served.

For example, prior to the establishment of regularly scheduled parent meetings, a group of parents may be asked to rate their satisfaction with the amount of information received from hospital personnel. Later, a group of parents who have participated in the meetings may complete the same evaluation form. A compilation of the responses received will indicate whether the goal of increasing parent satisfaction with access to information through parent meetings by the projected percentage was achieved.

An Outside Observer

Someone, such as a child life worker from another hospital or other professional, may be invited to study the functioning of the child life program, or a portion thereof, and complete a written evaluation form. For example, the evaluation mechanism of a proposal to obtain funds for the establishment of an adolescent lounge may consist of an assessment of the completed area by a recognized expert in the field.

Statistical Data

Statistics compiled with the assistance of the medical records department or through one's own record keeping may be used as another form of evaluation. For example, a child life department may be able to show that by increasing the play opportunities of children or by instituting a preoperative preparation program, children recuperate more quickly. Therefore, the statistics for a group of patients with a given condition, such as tonsillectomy surgery, who have not had access to these services may be compared with a similar group who participated in the newly instituted program. An analysis of the data may reveal that those children having access to the additional child life service had a significantly shorter hospital stay.

A review of statistical data from the patients' medical records may reveal other trends. For example, the amount of time between admissions for patients with chronic conditions such as asthma may increase following the institution of child life services. The number of patients using the outpatient clinic may rise, or a decline in missed appointments may be noted, following the establishment of a playroom in that department.

Data of this nature may be beneficial in monitoring the effects of the implementation of child life programming when used in combination with other forms of evaluation. It is unwise, however, to use measurements of this sort as a sole means of evaluation of programs. These figures are dependent on a large number of variables, few of which are readily controllable. For example, increased utilization of medical services may be more easily traced to seasonal health cycles, and missed appointments may be caused by a temporary transit strike. Furthermore, it is difficult at times to predict the possible positive effects of the introduction of new services. It may be anticipated that an outpatient child life program will increase the number of total patient visits, for instance, but instead the number declines due to parents' increased attention to nutrition, safety, and preventative medicine—subjects they learned about through the parent education component of the outpatient child life program.

Other forms of statistics may prove more reliable in demonstrating program value. These figures, which may be compiled by the child life staff, detail the extent of the services offered by the department and the number of people making use of them. Statistics such as the total number of patient contacts per given period of time, number of children participating in playroom activities or special events, or number of children and parents prepared for surgery, may be tabulated to indicate the level of child life activity. Information of this sort may also be used to measure the effectiveness of instituting new services. For example, the number of parents per month who "room in" with their children can be recorded prior to and following the institution of daily parent orientation meetings, to see if these gatherings are useful in encouraging more parents to stay.

Behavioral Ratings

Ratings of behavior may be used to determine the effectiveness of child life programming in minimizing the negative effects of hospitalization. A primary objective of many child life interventions such as therapeutic play sessions, preoperative teaching, and parent discussion groups is the reduction of fears, stress, and anxiety experienced by hospitalized children and their parents. One way of demonstrating success in achieving this goal is to observe the actions of children and parents who have participated in available programming and compare them with the behavior of those who have not. A reduction in the level of behaviors generally associated with psychological upset among those receiving child life services indicates the effectiveness of the intervention. A study may show, for example, that 50 percent of the children who did not participate in a preadmission tour experienced sleep disturbances in the hospital, while only 5 percent of those taking the tour had any difficulty.

For this method of evaluation to be of use in comparing groups of patients or parents, a standardized form, or behavioral rating scale, must be developed, with criteria for categorizing the various behaviors observed. Wolfer and Visintainer (1975), for example, developed two simple behavioral rating scales for determining the effectiveness of their method of preparation for surgery: a manifest upset scale and a cooperation scale. The manifest upset scale was a five-point scale designed to reflect the child's emotional state at the time of observation:

> A rating of one indicates little or no fear or anxiety (calm appearance, no crying, no verbal protest). A rating of three, a moderate amount (some temporary whimpering and/or mild verbal protest), and a rating of five indicates extreme emotional distress (agitated, hard crying or screaming and/or strong verbal protest) (p. 249).

The cooperation scale, also a five-point scale, indicates the child's degree of cooperation observable during the performance of a procedure:

> A rating of one indicates complete cooperation including active participation in and assistance with the procedure. A rating of three indicates mild or initial resistance or passive participation without assistance. A rating of five indicates extreme resistance, strong avoidance, and the necessity to restrain the child (p. 249).

Using these scales, an independent observer, who did not know which children had participated in the preparation sessions, observed the children at various stressful points during the hospitalization. The results of these observations, in conjunction with other measures, enabled the researchers to assess the value of the preparation process. Child life workers wishing to demonstrate the effectiveness of preparation for surgery or medical procedures or the value of medical play sessions may devise similar rating scales.

The type of behavior evaluated by the rating scale is determined by the stated objective of the service being evaluated. Thus, while the effectiveness of a preparation program may be evaluated by observation of the child's protest behavior or participation in procedures, the value of providing playroom activities might be measured by the amount of time children spend in active play, as opposed to idleness or inappropriate activities.

For example, an outpatient playroom may be established, in part, to reduce the incidence of behavior that the staff considers dangerous or disruptive, e.g. playing in ashtrays, climbing bookcases, or running in crowded areas. The rating scale devised by the child life staff to evaluate the effect of the play program must reflect the frequency with which children engage in various behaviors or the amount of time devoted to each activity. The scale should be applied before the program is started, and again after its institution to determine its effectiveness in altering the quality of the activities in which children engage.

Behavioral rating scales may also be modified for use in determining the emotional state of parents and the effects of programming on its improvement. An independent observer may apply such scales, noting the parents' verbal responses and nonverbal behaviors, much the same as with children. In other cases, a form of self-report by parents may be employed. Skipper and Leonard (1968), for example, had parents complete a questionnaire asking their perceptions of their own stress, confidence in medical personnel, and desire for information. Mechanisms of this sort are helpful in determining the effectiveness of providing parents with preparation, emotional support, and increased information during hospitalization.

The value of in-hospital interventions on the post-hospital adjustment of children and parents may also be determined by a rating of observable behaviors. Parents may be asked to complete a questionnaire concerning the behavior of their children following discharge. A simple five-point scale, similar to those employed by Wolfer and Visintainer (1975), could be designed to assess post-hospital patterns in sleeping, eating, toilet-training, and clinging to parents—areas in which problems are frequently noticed. When evaluating sleeping habits, for example, a rating of one might indicate that the child goes to sleep with no greater difficulty than prior to hospitalization. A rating of three might mean occasional or moderate sleeping disturbances, such as temporary crying before sleep; while five would indicate severe sleep disturbance, such as terrified crying and the child's refusal to sleep unless parents are present.

Some researchers have used the Post-hospital Behavior Questionnaire (formulated by Vernon et al, 1966) as a way of measuring the post-hospital responses of children. Parents may also be asked to complete a self-report form indicating their own responses following discharge. By using these instruments to compare the responses of individuals receiving specified child life services with those who have not, the child life staff can determine the effectiveness of programming in reducing post-hospital upset.

Physiological Measures

Instead of, or in addition to, using self-report indicators of upset or even the ratings of observers, both of which are "indirect," physiological indicators such as pulse rates, blood pressure and temperature may be used as measures of the level of stress present in children. According to Skipper and Leonard (1968), "Children at this age (3 to 9 years) have not developed effective inhibiting mechanisms, so that an increase in excitement, apprehension, anxiety and fear, etc., will be reflected in the level of these indicators (p. 279)." Thus, by measuring these variables an approximation of the child's emotional state can be obtained. These measurements are easily acquired, since they are routinely monitored by the nursing staff, and they have the added benefit of being objective. Whereas the behavioral ratings are subject to the interpretation of the observer, physiological measures, obtained by recording data obtained with the use of instruments, are not. Using these measures one can determine the effectiveness of an intervention in reducing stress in children. For example, the vital signs of children might be taken following an EKG procedure, to compare those of children who have and have not had an opportunity to play through the event prior to its occurrence.

Researchers have frequently used other quantifiable data related to physiological processes as indicators of the emotional state of children. Wolfer and Visintainer (1975) recorded the ease of fluid intake and the time to first voiding of children following surgery, as well as the patient's need for postoperative pain medication. Children who are less upset following surgery tend to take fluids with greater ease, urinate sooner, and be in less need of calming medications than those who are highly agitated. Thus, when a child life worker is seeking to demonstrate the effectiveness of preparation or preoperative play sessions in calming children postoperatively, measurements of this sort may be used in the analysis.

COST/BENEFIT ANALYSIS

In certain situations, it may be advantageous for the child life department to submit a cost/benefit analysis as an addendum to the program proposal. This type of analysis, frequently used by companies as a means of evaluating the merits of an investment, compares the monetary value of the benefits derived from an investment with the costs entailed by the project.

While it is difficult to place a monetary value on the benefits of child life programming (and some may object to attempts to do so), the efforts may be worthwhile. Child life programs, as a rule, do not generate income as do other hospital specialties, and therefore they are frequently in a weaker position when competing for scarce hospital dollars with departments that "pay their own way." Through a cost/benefit analysis, child life workers can demonstrate the value of the service to the hospital and the community, thereby permitting individuals in decision-making capacities to view the worth of seemingly intangible, yet invaluable, services from a financial perspective.

Steps in a Cost/Benefit Analysis

When preparing a cost/benefit analysis, the child life staff must first describe the expected benefits of instituting the program in question. The stated benefits should be quite specific and capable of being translated into monetary value. For example, benefits from the institution of a preparation program might be the increased cooperation of children during medical procedures, a reduction in post-hospital psychological upset, and increased utilization of the pediatric facilities due to the satisfaction of pediatricians and families.

After listing the expected benefits, these items must be converted into monetary value. A portion of the benefits, termed *cost avoidance* benefits, represents savings anticipated as a result of the program. In the case of a preparation program, the increased cooperation of children with procedures reduces the amount of staff time spent in their administration, and therefore results in cost avoidance savings for the hospital.

Another portion of the cost avoidance benefits will accrue to the families of children who, due to the preparation program, will not need to avail themselves of psychiatric or counseling services. Numerous studies have shown that a substantial percentage of children who are not prepared for hospitalization and surgery suffer long-term psychological upset. This number is greatly reduced among children who have had adequate preparation. Based on these studies and on the number of pediatric surgeries performed at the facility, an estimate of the number of children who are annually spared the necessity for additional professional help can be made. A monetary value for these benefits can be derived by multiplying this theoretical number by an average cost of therapy, arrived at in consultation with psychiatric personnel.

In addition to cost avoidance benefits, the hospital and the children served also receive benefits in the form of *return on investment.* The hospital, for example, can be expected to receive additional income due to the increased utilization of the pediatric facility. Children who avoid psychological problems as a result of the preparation program have an increased capacity to become productive adults. The expected increase in hospital revenue, and the anticipated future incomes of the children, which may have been diminished or eliminated by incapacitating emotional problems, may be included in the return on investment benefits.

Cost estimates must reflect the total costs of running the program over a period of time. Initial investments for furnishings, equipment and construction, as well as annual operating costs (salaries, fringe benefits, consumable supplies, and overhead) are included in the estimate. Finally, the estimated monetary value of seemingly free resources, such as volunteer labor and donated materials, is added to other costs.

When computing the cost/benefit ratio of a proposed program, the expected future benefits are "discounted" by a set amount, commonly 10 percent. This adjustment accounts for the fact that the money spent on the program might be devoted to another investment from which earnings of a certain amount can reasonably be expected. Thus, the proposed program benefits must be shown to be in excess of the amount reasonably expected from other investments.

The cost/benefit ratio, then, is calculated in this manner:

$$\frac{\text{Discounted cost avoidance savings} + \text{discounted return on investment}}{\text{initial investment} + \text{operating costs}}$$

A ratio of greater than one demonstrates that the benefits exceed the costs, while a ratio of less than one shows the opposite. For example, a proposed program with a ratio of 2.5 would be a better investment, all other things being equal, than a program with a cost/benefit ratio of only .3.

Sample Cost/Benefit Analysis

A cost/benefit analysis for a comprehensive preparation program serving a 20-bed pediatric unit might be completed in this manner. Of the 1500 annual pediatric admissions, 500 surgeries are performed. A conservative estimate is made that one percent of the children, or five children, would likely suffer long-term psychological upset, preventable through the preparation program. The average cost of therapy for these children is estimated at $500. Therefore, cost avoidance for the family would equal $2500.

Estimates further indicate that the increase cooperation of patients will reduce the amount of staff time spent administering medications and procedures and restraining reluctant children, not only in the pediatric unit, but in surgery, X-ray, the laboratory, and other areas. This time is approximately equal to that of one full-time staff person; therefore, cost avoidance for the hospital equals $20,000.

The total cost avoidance figure is $22,500—or, when discounted by 10 percent, $20,250.

The return on investment to the hospital due to increased utilization is expected to be a relatively modest $2,000 for the first year, but is expected to increase thereafter. Thus, for the first year of operation, the return on investment for the hospital is $2,000.

Of the five children who can be expected to suffer long-term emotional upset without benefit of the preparation program, it is estimated that these problems will substantially impair the potential future income of two of them. With an average potential future income of $500,000 for each, a 25 percent reduction in this amount, attributable to the disability, would total $125,000. Since the presence of the preparation program would have prevented the psychological upset, thereby allowing each child to earn this extra amount, the return on investment to children equals $250,000.

The total return on investment figure is $252,000—or, when discounted by 10 percent, $226,800.

Costs for the program are budgeted as follows:

Initial Investment	
Equipment	$1,000
Furnishings	500
TOTAL	$1,500
Operating Costs	
Personnel	$17,000
Fringe Benefits	3,000
Consumable Equipment	1,000
Overhead	2,000
TOTAL	$23,000

Total costs for the first year of operation equal $24,500.

Using the formula for deriving the cost/benefit ratio, the discounted cost avoidance benefits of $20,250 are added to the discounted return on investment benefits of $226,800 to equal $247,050 in total benefits. This total is divided by total costs of the program for the first year of operation, or

$$\frac{\text{Total Discounted Benefits}}{\text{Total Costs}} \text{ equals } \frac{\$247,050}{24,500} \text{ equals greater than } \frac{10}{1}$$

Thus, the estimate of costs to benefits for the first year of operation is in excess of 10 to 1, a highly favorable ratio, indicating the value of the investment.

It is impossible to place an acceptable value on the benefit of an emotionally sound child to a parent or a child's capacity to attain adulthood unfettered by lingering psychological problems. One can, however, through the mechanism of a cost/benefit analysis, begin to examine some of the "hidden" benefits society gains through the implementation of child life programming. In financial terms, a modest investment of time and resources in the establishment of these services returns substantial benefits to the hospital providing them, to the families participating in them, and to the community as a whole.

INCREASING SUPPORT FOR CHILD LIFE PROGRAMMING

Any proposal for the introduction of child life programming, for the expansion of services offered, or the alteration of unacceptable conditions in the environment will be looked upon more favorably if presented with the support of hospital personnel and the consumers using the facility. For this reason child life personnel should be aware of mechanisms they may use to encourage that support in order to cultivate a proper climate for initiating change.

Support of Hospital Personnel

In Chapter 7, it was proposed that resistance to child life programming arising from disciplines within the hospital might be reduced through the use of several forms of intervention. Among these interventions are the use of education, personal preparedness, cooperation with other professionals, and offering services that meet the needs of others. Even as these interventions are useful in reducing the amount of resistance encountered by child life workers, so are they helpful in encouraging support for child life programming among individuals who, though not resistant, are also not enthusiastic.

Through educational activities, the child life staff can promote the goals of the department, while at the same time offering helpful insights to hospital personnel that will assist them in their interactions with children. For example, an inservice provided for laboratory personnel may be used to inform them of the value of needle play and preparation for children, in addition to offering specific suggestions for approaching children of various ages when drawing blood. The inservice offers specific help to the laboratory workers, thereby demonstrating the willingness of child life personnel to cooperate with other disciplines, while also providing a forum for the further promotion of child life objectives. Laboratory personnel who have benefitted from this educational experience and are knowledgeable about the needs of children are likely to support the continuation or expansion of child life services.

At times, support for child life programming is lacking merely because of the limited number of people in the hospital who know if its existence or function. In such cases efforts must be made to increase the visibility of the services offered. For example, some of the stated annual objectives for child life may lend themselve to a project in which all hospital personnel may participate. This might consist of increasing the amount of materials donated to the playroom by having employees save certain items from home. The collection campaign may be publicized throughout the hospital, with a depository being in or near the playroom. Therefore, when the cardboard tubes and plastic bottles are lugged to the area, the employees have an opportunity to view child life activities in progress.

Hospital personnel may also be polled to discover the talents they possess that children never see. Undoubtedly, a number of singers, painters, guitar players, and woodcrafters will be found. These individuals may be asked to donate their time occasionally to entertain or work with children on specific projects. Not only does this process familiarize the employees with child life services and allow them a place in the implementation, it also permits children to view the staff out of the role of doctor, nurse, or laboratory technician.

The child life staff may also raise the visibility of its programming by doing a research project on a given subject; the effects of 24-hour visitation for parents, for example. As Finkel (no date) has pointed out, in the course of running a pilot project on an element of programming that may be controversial to some interest is stirred, people participate, become aware of the conditions existing in the pediatric unit, and may decide that they like the innovation being studied, regardless of the statistical outcome.

The most successful way of increasing the visibility of the child life program is through use of the media. The pediatric unit and child life programming provide unlimited material for newspaper and magazine articles, television and radio interviews, and public service announcements. Through these vehicles the objectives of child life programming can be widely disseminated, raising the profile of the program within the hospital and throughout the community.

Support of the Community

In addition to the support of other disciplines within the hospital, the child life staff should also pursue the support of members of the community in general. Through access to the media, such as newspaper articles or radio interviews, child life workers can begin to spread information to parents of the community, educating them concerning the types of services they may expect from their hospitals. Parent groups are frequently looking for speakers for their meetings and will welcome the presence of a hospital representative to discuss the care of hospitalized children.

By contracting community members through the media and in person, child life workers are helping to develop an informed group of consumers who are aware of the problems children face while hospitalized, and of the solutions available to help them. At times parents have formed groups to inform themselves about the hospitalization of children and to urge the implementation of appropriate changes. The visible support of a knowledgeable group of consumers will be very persuasive when child life workers propose changes for the benefit of hospitalized children

Appendices

CHILD LIFE ACTIVITY STUDY
SECTION POSITION PAPER*

Child Life Programs in health care settings strive to promote optimum development of children, adolescents and families, to maintain normal living patterns and to minimize psychological trauma. As integral members of the health care team in both the ambulatory care and inpatient settings, child life staff provide opportunities for gaining a sense of mastery, for play, for learning, for self-expression, for family involvement and for peer interaction.

I. RATIONALE FOR CHILD LIFE PROGRAMS
- Excessive anxiety and stress related to illness, separation, hospitalization, and medical encounters can be emotionally damaging to an infant, child or adolescent as well as interfere with his or her optimal response to medical treatment and care.
- Major interruptions of normal life experiences can jeopardize growth and development.
- Physical limitations of illness and hospitalization invite dependency and can erode self-esteem.
- Compared to the general population, children and adolescents in health care settings are more likely to have previously experienced excessive social, familial and environmental stress.
- A child's hospitalization can at times be a positive growth experience when truly comprehensive care is given. Such comprehensive care by definition includes child life services staffed by appropriately trained personnel. These services are derived from the ACCH policy statement with a particular focus on the following:

II. ESSENTIAL GOALS OF CHILD LIFE PROGRAMS
A. Minimizing stress and anxiety for the child, and adolescent
1. Provide abundant play opportunities and other experiences which encourage expression of feelings and promote a sense of mastery and understanding of medical experiences. This necessitates qualified personnel, provision of suitable play materials and opportunities for medical play.

---

*From the Association for the Care of Children in Hospitals.

2. Increase the familiarity of surroundings and events by encouraging, supporting, or providing:
   (a) within the community, programs to acquaint children with the hospital
   (b) preadmission orientation visits
   (c) informational materials for children, adolescents, and parents
   (d) familiarization of the child with new surroundings upon admission
   (e) explanations comprehensible to the child of the sequence, nature and reasons for procedures and routines, as well as the presence of a supportive individual
   (f) a physical environment that is appropriate and receptive to the age-groups exposed to it
3. Maintain the child's relationship with parents and other family members.
   (a) promote policies which encourage unrestricted parental visiting, rooming-in, and parental presence during stressful events
   (b) provide opportunities for parents to actively continue their parenting role
   (c) communicate with parents about their child's feelings and behavior and extend support to parents with an understanding of their own stress and needs
   (d) provide opportunities for sibling and peer visiting
4. Provide supportive relationship for patients and parents characterized by warmth, empathy, respect and understanding of developmental stages.

B. **Provision of Essential Life Experiences**
   1. Provide play opportunities and other experiences which foster continued growth and development and prevent adverse reactions to hospitalization.
   2. Provide home-like activities such as cooking, outdoor play, and eating in groups.
   3. Encourage an active school program in the hospital with qualified teaching personnel and classroom facilities.
   4. Screen interested groups in the community who wish to be involved in activities for children and interpret child life activity programs and needs of pediatric patients to them.

C. **Providing Opportunities to Retain Self-Esteem and Appropriate Independence**
   1. Ensure recognition of the child as a unique individual.
   2. Encourage inclusion of patients in decision making to a degree consistent with their level of development.
   3. Foster responsibility for self and others.

4. Provide access to equipment and facilities that encourages maximum independence, minimizing loss of competency, and enhances the rehabilitative process.
5. Heighten feelings of competency by providing opportunities to be creative and successful at a variety of experiences.

III. **STANDARDS FOR PERSONNEL**

    A. **Child Life Specialist**

    Academic preparation at the Bachelor's Degree level with supervised experience in the health care setting and competence in the following areas: growth and development, family dynamics, play and activities, interpersonal communication, developmental observation and assessment, the learning process, group process, behavior management, the reactions of children to hospitalization and to illness, interventions to prevent emotional trauma, collaboration with other health care professionals, basic understanding of children's illnesses and medical terminology, supervisory skills.

    B. **Child Life Assistant**

    Such a person (to work only under the direct supervision of a Child Life Specialist) would generally hold a diploma in an appropriately related field and have personal qualifications similar to the above.

    C. **Child Life Administrator**

    Academic preparation at the Master's Degree level contributing to expertise in all of the areas listed under Child Life Specialist. In addition, it is necessary for the administrator to be competent in: establishing program objectives, interpreting objectives and needs to Child Life staff, administration within the hospital system, selecting, supervising and evaluating staff, managing budget and organizing resources to provide most effective service, providing educational resources regarding child life needs to students, other staff and the community, maintaining good interdepartmental communication as well as keeping abreast of related programs in health care settings and other associated organizations.

IV. **ADMINISTRATION OF PROGRAM**

    The Child Life Program should be autonomous, having an equal status with other departments, and report directly to the Administrator.

    The minimum child life specialist-to-child ratio should be 1 to 10: this includes basic coverage for days, evenings, weekends and holidays. Funding for staff, developmentally appropriate materials, equipment and activities should be a part of the regular hospital budget and not dependent on donations.

    Communication with other health care staff must include:

(a) sensitivity to team process and awareness of roles and expertise of other health professionals;

(b) reciprocal sharing of information pertinent to the medical and psychosocial needs of children and families;

(c) inservice education for hospital staff on the various needs of children, adolescents, and their families;

(d) communication of observations, assessments, and recommendations for care in the form of daily verbal reports, multidisciplinary rounds and recording on patients' records.

The Child Life Program should utilize the institutional charting system and format.

Adequate space, equipment, materials and personnel should be allocated to the Child Life Program to ensure that patients will be provided with safe, therapeutic, enriching and appropriately stimulating play and learning areas readily accessible to children and adolescents.

Responsibility for training and supervising volunteers and students participating in the Child Life Program should be assumed by Child Life personnel.

Departmental policies and procedures shall be in compliance with the overall institutional policies and procedures currently in existence.

The Child Life Director should conduct a periodic assessment of the quality and appropriateness of care provided by the Child Life staff and provide for continuing staff education and development.

Approved Summer 1979
Association for the Care
of Children in Hospitals
3615 Wisconsin Avenue
Washington, D.C. 20016

APPENDIX B

POSITION STATEMENT ON INVOLVEMENT OF PARENTS AND FAMILIES IN HEALTH CARE SETTINGS*

I. PHILOSOPHY

Children are both individuals and members of the family. Medical care, acute or chronic, creates varying degrees of stress on a family unit (Vernon, et. al., 1965.) Since the health care system influences the child and the family, care involves the entire "family."

This position paper presents the general philosophy and goals espoused by the Association for the Care of Children in Hospitals in regard to parents and families. The general position taken in this paper is seen to apply to the wide range of health care settings, of staff situations and of economic conditions. Health care settings include hospitals and ambulatory settings regardless of size and function. Implementation of this philosophy necessitates individual and organizational decisions regarding involvement of parents and families. In providing for the care of parents and families, there are a number of concepts which are central for the organization of health care.

II. CENTRAL CONCEPTS

A. Maintenance of the tie between the child and family.

As Prugh (1953) stated in reviewing the emotional aspects of hospitalization on children, this continuation of the ties within the existing family unit is the most crucial aspect of meeting the mental health needs of the child in a health care facility. Maintaining the ties and bonds within the family preserves a major source of support for both the child and the family. Implementation can occur by a variety of activities. Examples might include: (1) rooming in, (2) providing varying degrees of physical care given by the parents either in the hospital or at home, (3) various visits by family members including siblings, (4) having pictures of family members, (5) encouraging telephone contacts. Regardless of the staffing patterns, the regulations of the particular health care

*From the Association for the Care of Children in Hospitals.

setting, or the capabilities of the individual family unit, *some* of these opportunities can be arranged which facilitate and strengthen family ties and bonds.

B. **Establishment of an environment where the child experiences a continued sense of parenting.**

Continuing parenting by the parents is of highest priority to the child and his family. When a "parent" cannot be present, the child needs to experience a stable relationship with a responsive person in order to maintain the "mothering attitude" (Robertson and Robertson, 1973; A. Freud, 1973; Heinicke, 1965; and Yarrow, 1964.) An awareness of the child's individual needs based upon the developmental stage and family experiences is an integral aspect of planning and implementing care for children and families. An understanding of these needs must be present in order to establish this continued "sense of parenting."

C. **Recognition of and respect for the means that the family has for adjusting and coping with the increased stress within the family system.**

Such recognition involves a determination of the support system and coping strategies that the family uses to meet stressful events. Chronic illness, acute illness and/or hospitalization cause a change in family interactions and result in varying degrees of stress for that family. The family unit should be involved in both long and short term planning for care when possible.

D. **Facilitation and support of the family's style of coping with stress.**

Coping styles of the family may be enhanced by: (1) providing families with continuing understandable information regarding the child's condition and therapies, (2) asking parents to provide information about "what works best at home with this child?", (3) discussing the child's and family's reaction to a contact with health care facility, (4) providing parent education through anticipatory counseling and involvement in planning for discharge and follow-up. Some styles may be counter-productive, perpetuating further stressful events and may not help the family arrive at a solution of the stress. These situations may require the health care provider to assist the family by means of various parent education techniques to develop or expand their coping repertoire.

E. **Management of conflict between family and health care systems.**

Various family styles may be in conflict with styles advocated by the health care facility. The health care provider must recognize conflict between the family system and the professional care system. All of the preceding concepts must be employed by the health care provider in seeking resolution of such conflict.

III. **RECOMMENDATIONS FOR IMPLEMENTATION**

Implementation of the above philosophy and concepts on the involvement of parents and families in the various health care settings requires our commitment. ACCH may assist individuals and institutions in this implementation by the following provisions:

A. Educational programs at both the central and local levels, particularly programs concerned with initiating change.

B. Consultation and resources that assist with implementation.

C. Input into official policy making groups, such as the Joint Commission, state licensing, and other units to develop standards of care.

D. Support of research to determine various modalities of care, to assess attitudes toward family centered care, and to develop tools that measure the effectiveness of new approaches to child care.

E. Development of standards of practice for individuals working with parents and families in health care settings, which involves assessment of the individual and the health care setting in which he works.

F. Stimulation of more publications in professional and non-professional journals regarding family involvement in the child's health care.

G. Maintenance of ties with parent and advocate groups.

POSITION STATEMENT ON THE CARE OF ADOLESCENTS AND FAMILIES IN HEALTH CARE SETTINGS*

"... neither the human body nor the mind, neither the intellect nor the emotions are separate entities which function independently of each other; on the contrary, they are linked by ties which if neglected endanger the individual ... "

Anna Freud[1]

PREAMBLE

There has been a growing awareness in the health care community that the needs of adolescents in modern society must be met by efforts directed at specific stages in the adolescent's life. Traditionally, medicine has dealt with the adolescent as belonging to the "adult world." No longer can we yield to the argument that the adolescent represents merely a younger adult, nor can we casually consider the adolescent still a child.

Increasing medical knowledge has permitted more ill children and adolescents to live, and in most cases, to live more fully. The physical requirements and inner psychic demands of this age-group make the care of the adolescent a complex and challenging task, thus creating the need for specialized services.

There is more to learn about the effects of illness, treatment, and health care settings on the emotional development of adolescent patients. However, sufficient knowledge now exists to direct action toward both minimizing psychological damage and promoting coping abilities. Research, communication among professionals, appropriate parent involvement, and greater understanding of the emotional life of adolescents, are essential to provide for the cognitive, psychosocial, medical, and environmental needs of this special group of patients.

I. PHILOSOPHY

This position paper presents the general philosophy and goals espoused by the Association for the Care of Children's Health in regard to the care of adolescents in health care settings. It attempts

---

*From the Association for the Care of Children's Health.

256

to identify the needs, responsibilities and rights of adolescent patients, of their families and of the staff working with them. Implementation of this philosophy necessitates individual and institutional commitment to the care of adolescents.

The Association for the Care of Children's Health endorses the following policies:

A. **That all health care settings serving adolescents should:**
   1. Be prepared to offer comprehensive management of the adolescent patient based on an understanding of adolescent development as well as medical needs.
   2. Provide in-patient services which meet the requirements of the Guidelines for Adolescent Units set out by the Association for the Care of Children's Health.
   3. Have available a written philosophy of adolescent care, which acknowledges the unique needs of adolescents. The statement should be available to and readily understood by patients and families.

B. **That for every adolescent patient:**
   1. The rights to confidentiality and consent be recognized. Current trends in case and statutory law, as reflected by the Supreme Court of the United States ruling in 1976,[2] afirm that adolescents are indeed individuals with their own right to decision making and confidentiality. While it is usually best to work toward including the parents in medical decisions, adolescents are often in need of obtaining confidential health care on their own consent. When in the judgement of the health care professional treatment is deemed necessary for the adolescent's benefit, and when it is fully understood and appropriately consented to by the patient, treatment should be allowed with or without parental consent. This situation applies particularly in relation to venereal disease, pregnancy, alcohol and drug abuse, psychiatric difficulties, and other conditions which have specific meaning to adolescents. Laws relating to these issues vary between each state and each province.[3] Adolescents and families should have available information on local laws as well as specific hospital policies on minor's rights.
   2. Health education programs be provided to promote adolescents' understanding and mastery of body and illness.
   3. Educational needs be met by provision of appropriate school programs for both in and out-patients. This will involve vocational guidance and liaison with the general educational system.
   4. Social, emotional and recreational needs be recognized, and opportunities provided for the ill adolescent to meet normal developmental tasks while in the hospital, school, community,

and with peers and family.
5. Responsibility with regard to self-care and decision-making be identified and promoted.
6. The individual's coping mechanisms be respected and receive appropriate response by staff.

C. **That for the family of the adolescent patient:**
1. There be encouragement of a continuing relationship with the patient.
2. There be recognition of the right of information, visiting, and appropriate inclusion in the adolescent's health care, while encouraging the family to support the adolescent's need for independence, confidentiality, and decision making.
3. Attention be given to cultural, religious, and environmental influences upon families' responses to illness and treatment.
4. There be provided education and psychosocial support in dealing with the illness and health care of the adolescent.

D. **That the staff:**
1. Respect and respond appropriately to the developmental needs of adolescents.
2. Be selected and trained specifically to work with adolescents.
3. Establish a mechanism for interdisciplinary communication and coordination of services.
4. Have a formal program of continuing education.
5. Provide both in and out-patient health education on subjects related to diseases and to health maintenance.
6. Promote research into health problems of and services to adolescents.
7. Develop instructive and participatory seminars for the community in order to disseminate information on diseases and health maintenance of adolescents.
8. Develop ambulatory services and support programs whenever possible.

II. **RECOMMENDATIONS FOR IMPLEMENTATION**
We urge each hospital to make an institutional commitment to the care of adolescents by establishing a standing committee with function and accountability defined in writing. The committee:
1. Is responsible for developing a written philosophy on adolescent care.
2. Sets policies and procedures, based on pertinent local laws, for the minor and the family regarding confidentiality, release of health information, payment, referral to low-cost or free facilities, emergency services, and minor's eligibility to consent.
3. Reviews periodically the policies mentioned above, considering recent precedents, changes in laws, and trends in minor's rights.

4. Provides policy statements as deemed necessary regarding conditions and procedures such as pregnancies, or amputations, which have a special meaning to adolescents.
5. Promotes research.
6. Provides coordination of continuing education.
7. Is available for consultation by the staff working with adolescents.

Each committee should be composed of members of the medical, administrative, and supportive disciplines familiar with adolescents' care with consideration given to lawyer and parent and youth representatives sitting on the committee.

III. THE ROLE OF ACCH IN IMPLEMENTATION

ACCH should support individuals and institutions in their endeavors by:

1. Disseminating standards of practice for adolescent care.
2. Developing lines of communication with other organizations interested in or caring for adolescents.
3. Promoting information and research.
4. Keeping up with new trends in adolescent care and up-dating this statement as needed.

References:
1. From Anna Freud's Foreword to "The Hospitalized Adolescent" by Hoffman, A. D., Becker, R. D. Gabriel, H R., The Free Press, 1976.
2. Planned Parenthood of Central Missouri vs. Danforth 74-1151 (1976).
3. Specific information on laws for legal rights of minors can be obtained in the U.S. from the state's attorney general, local departments of health and planned parenthood offices, and in Canada from the Federal and provincial departments of justice.

For more information:
"Survey of Activity Programs for Hospitalized Adolescents and Annotated Bibliography", ACCH 1977. "Guidelines for Adolescent Units," in Proceedings from Washington, D.C. Conference, ACCH 1978.

Approved June 1979
Association for the
Care of Children's Health
3615 Wisconsin Avenue
Washington, D.C. 20016
(202) 244-1801

STATEMENTS OF POLICY
FOR THE CARE OF CHILDREN
AND FAMILIES IN HEALTH CARE SETTINGS*

Preamble

Advancement of technology and medical science has permitted more children to live, to live longer and in most cases, to live more fully. In the process, other dangers to children's healthy development have arisen or come to light. These problems have in turn stimulated the current progress in the behavioral sciences.

Threats posed to the emotional security and development of many children and their families by serious illness, disability, disfigurement, treatment, interrupted human relationships and nonsupportive environments have been clearly demonstrated by worldwide research studies. The outcomes can range from temporary but frequently overwhelming anxiety and emotional suffering to long-standing or permanent developmental handicaps. Such interference with the fullest possible development and expression of individual potential is an unacceptable price to pay.

Closer contact with the emotional life of children, increased parent involvement and communication amongst professionals have also contributed to greater understanding as well as to improvements of care. Whereas there is still much to learn regarding the inter-relatedness of such factors as age, type of illness, length of hospitalization, critical developmental periods and vulnerability, sufficient knowledge now exists to direct action toward both minimizing and preventing such harm.

The Association for the Care of Children in Hospitals endorses the following policies:

All pediatric health care settings should:

1. have a stated philosophy of care which is specific, easily understood by, and made available to patients and families, and which applies in a coordinated manner to all disciplines and departments.
2. Assist or provide programs of prevention and restorative care which respond to emotional, social and environmental causal factors of accidents and illness.

---

*From the Association for the Care of Children in Hospitals

3. Create and maintain a social and physical environment which is as welcoming, unthreatening and supportive as possible, and which fosters open communication, encourages human relationships, and invites involvement of children, their families and the community in decisions affecting their care.
4. Avoid hospitalizing children whenever possible through the development of alternatives.
5. Develop and utilize ambulatory, day and home care programs which are financially and geographically accessible.
6. Minimize the duration of unavoidable hospital stays, while recognizing discharge planning needs.
7. Provide for and encourage the presence and participation in the hospital of persons most significant to the child, to approximate supportive home patterns of interactions and routines.
8. Provide consistent, emotionally supportive nurturing care for young children during the absence of their parents.
9. Respect the unique care-taking role of parents as well as their individual responses, and provide ongoing understandable information and support which will enable them to utilize their strengths in supporting their child.
10. Provide a milieu which is responsive to the uniqueness of each child and adolescent, their ethnic and cultural backgrounds and developmental needs.
11. Provide readily accessible, well designed space, equipment and programs for the wide range of play, educational and social activities which are essential to all children and adolescents, particularly those who have been deprived of normal opportunities for development.
12. Provide child care professionals who are skilled at assessing emotional, developmental and academic needs, communicating with and fostering the involvement of patients and their families in activities appropriate to their needs.
13. Ensure that children and their parents are informed, understand and are supported prior to, during, and following experiences which are potentially distressing.
14. Carefully select all staff and volunteers according to their commitment to the foregoing policies. Those in direct contact, however limited, with children, youth, and families should be sensitive, perceptive, and compassionate. Professionals involved in more extended, intimate, and responsible positions of child care should have special training in child development, family dynamics and the unique psychological needs of children when ill and under stress.
15. Facilitate orientation, continued learning, and consultation in relation to all of the above, and provide support which recognizes the emotional demands on staff.
16. Encourage and foster the inclusion of the above educational focus in

the basic curriculum and field experiences of the various professional and technical personnel preparing for careers in pediatric settings.

17. Support the evolvement of resources for early detection, and of attitudes and facilities for ongoing care of children with health and/or developmental problems.

18. Provide for ongoing evaluation of policies and programs by the recipients of care and staff at all levels.

19. Support and disseminate research which clarifies and pertains to the above.

20. Promote education within the community about the health and developmental needs of children.

REFERENCES

Altschuler, A. *Books That Help Children Deal with a Hospital Experience*. Washington, D.C.: U.S. Government Printing Office, 1978.

American Academy of Pediatrics, Committee on Hospital Care. *Care of Children in Hospitals*. (2nd ed.) Evanston, Illinois: AAP, 1971.

American Academy of Pediatrics, Committee on Hospital Care. *Hospital Care of Children and Youth*. Evanston, Illinois: AAP, 1978.

Association for the Care of Children in Hospitals. *Directory of Child Life Activity Programs in North America*. Washington, D.C.: ACCH, 1979.

Association for the Care of Children's Health. *Guidelines for the Development of Child Life Programs*. Washington, D.C.: ACCH, 1980.

Association for the Care of Children's Health, Child Life Activity Study Section. *Position Paper*. Washington, D.C.: ACCH, 1979.

Azarnoff, P. A play program in a pediatric clinic. *Children*. 1970, 17, 218–221.

Azarnoff, P., & Flegal, S. *A Pediatric Play Program: Developing Therapeutic Play Programs for Children in Medical Settings*. Springfield, Illinois: Charles C Thomas, 1975.

Barnett, C., Leiderman, H., Grobstein, R., & Klaus, M. Neonatal separation: The maternal side of deprivation, *Pediatrics*, 1970, 45, 197.

Bolles, R. N. *What Color is Your Parachute? A Practical Manual for Job-hunters and Career-changers*. Berkeley: Ten Speed Press, 1978.

Bowlby, J. Separation anxiety. *International Journal of Psychoanalysis*, 1960, 41, 89–113.

Burton, L. *The Family Life of Sick Children*. Boston: Routledge & Kegan Paul, 1975.

Campbell, E. II. Effects of mothers' anxiety on infants' behavior. Unpublished doctoral dissertation, Yale University, 1957.

Casler, L. Maternal deprivation: A critical review of the literature. *Monographs of the Society for Research in Child Development*, 1961 26(2).

Crocker, E. *Child Life Programs in the Maritime Provinces: A Study of the Medical Needs of and Future Directions for Hospitalized Children*. Halifax: Atlantic Institute of Education, 1974.

Douglas, J. W. B. Early hospital admissions and later disturbances of behavior and learning. *Developmental Medicine and Child Neurology*, 1975, 17, 456–480.

Eckenhoff, J. E. Relationship of anesthesia to postoperative personality changes in children. *American Journal of Disabled Children*, 1953, 86, 587–591.

Erickson, F. Play interviews for four-year-old hospitalized children. Monographs of the *Society for Research in Child Development*, 1958, 23(3).

Erikson, E. H. *Childhood and Society*. New York: Norton, 1963.

Family Communications. *Let's Talk About the Hospital: A Guide for Hospital Staff*. Pittsburgh: Family Communications, 1977.

Fassler, D. Reducing preoperative anxiety in children: Information versus emotional support. Paper presented at annual meeting of the American Orthopsychiatric Association, Washington, D.C., 1979.

Finkel, K. C. Hospital politics and change: The art of the sometime possible. In Association for the Care of Children in Hospitals, *Human Needs and Political Realities*. Washington, D.C.: ACCH, no date.

Flavell, J. H. *The Developmental Psychology of Jean Piaget*. New York: D. Van Nostrand, 1963.

Freud, A. The role of bodily illness in the mental life of children. In R. Eissler et al. (Eds.), *Physical Illness and Handicap in Childhood*. New Haven: Yale University Press, 1977.

Garvey, C. *Play*. Cambridge: Harvard University Press, 1977.

Gofman, H., Buckman, W., & Schade, G. H. Parents' emotional response to child's hospitalization. *American Journal of the Diseases of Children*, 1957, 93, 629–637.

Hardgrove, C. Children respond to therapeutic art. *Hospitals*, April 16, 1980, 67–69.

Hardgrove, C. Helping parents on the pediatric ward: A report on a survey of hospitals with "living-in" programs. *Paediatrician*, 1980 9, 220-223.

Hardgrove, C. What every parent needs to know about rooming-in. Unpublished paper, no date.

Hardgrove, C. Working with parents on the pediatric unit. *Pediatric Annals*, 1972, 1(3), 44–62.

Hardgrove, C., & Dawson, R. *Parents and Children in the Hospital*. Boston: Little, Brown, 1972.

Hardgrove, C., & Rutledge, A. Parenting during hospitalization. *American Journal of Nursing*, 1975, 75, 836–838.

Hartley, R. E., & Goldenson, R. M. *The Complete Book of Children's Play*. New York: Thomas Y. Crowell, 1963.

Hofmann, A. D., Becker, R. D., & Gabriel, H. P. *The Hospitalized Adolescent*. New York: The Free Press, 1976.

Howells, J. G., & Layng, J. The effect of separation experiences on children given care away from home. *Medical Officer*, 1956, 95(26), 334–345.

Jackson, K., Winkley, R., Faust, O. A., Cermak, E. G., & Burtt, M. M. Behavior changes indicating emotional trauma in tonsillectomized children. *Pediatrics*, 1953, 12, 23–27.

Jacoby, N. M. Unrestricted visiting in a children's ward. *Lancet*, 1969, 47, 548–586.

James, F. E. The behavior reactions of normal children to common operations. *Practitioner*, 1960, 185, 339–342.

Jessner, L., Bloom, G. D., & Waldfogel, S. Emotional implications of tonsillectomy and adenoidectomy on children. In R. S. Eissler et al. (Eds.), *Physical Illness and Handicap in Childhood*. New Haven: Yale University Press, 1977.

Johnson, B. H. Before hospitalization: A preparation program for the child and his family. *Children Today*, 1974, 87, 18–21.

Johnson, J. E., Kirchhoff, K. T., & Endress, M. P. Altering children' distress behavior during orthopedic cast removal. *Nursing Research*, 1975, 24(6), 404–410.

Joint Commission on Mental Health in Children. *Crisis in child mental health — Challenge for the 70s*. New York: Harper & Row, 1971.

Kassowitz, K. E. Psychodynamic reactions of children to the use of hypodermic needles. *American Journal of the Diseases of Children*, 1958, 95, 253–257.

Kennell, J. H., Voos, D. K., & Klaus, M. H. Parent-infant bonding. In J. D. Osofsky (Ed.), *Handbook of Infant Development*. New York: Wiley, 1979.

Klinzing, D. R., & Klinzing, D. G. *The Hospitalized Child: Communication Techniques for Health Personnel*. Englewood Cliffs, New Jersey: Prentice-Hall, 1977.

Knight, J. Fair play for children. In Association for the Care of Children in Hospitals, *Human Needs and Political Realities*. Washington, D.C.: ACCH, no date.

Larsen, C. The child life professions: Today and tomorrow. In Association for the Care of Children's Health, *Child Life Activity*. Washington, D.C.: ACCH, no date.

Levy, D. M. Child patients may suffer psychic trauma after surgery. *Modern Hospital*, 1945, 65(6), 51–52.

Levy, D. M. The infant's earliest memory of innoculation: A contribution to public health procedures. *Journal of Genetic Psychology*, 1960, 96, 3–46.

Lindheim, R., Glaser, H. H., & Coffin, C. *Changing Hospital Environments for Children*. Cambridge: Harvard University Press, 1972.

Love, H. D., Henderson, S. K., & Stewart, M. K. *Your Child Goes to the Hospital: A Book for Parents*. Springfield, Illinois: Charles C Thomas, 1972.

Lowbury, E. J. L., & Jackson, D. M. Hospital infection and visitors. *British Medical Journal*, 1960, 1(5180), 1203–1204.

Marano, H., & Daniel, J. Children get better faster in homelike hospitals. *Family Weekly*, June 25, 1978, 14.

Mather, P. L., & Glasrud, P. H. Personal communication, June 29, 1980.

McCue, K., Wagner, M., Hansen, H., & Rigler, D. Survey of a developing health care profession: Hospital "play" programs. *Journal of the Association for the Care of Children in Hospitals*, 1978, 7(1), 15–22.

Melamed, B. G., & Siegel, L. J. Reduction of anxiety in children facing hospitalization and surgery by use of filmed modeling. *Journal of Consulting and Clinical Psychology*, 1975, 43, 511–521.

Moore, N. V., Evertson, D. J., & Brophy, J. E. Solitary play: Some functional reconsiderations. *Developmental Psychology*, 1974, 10, 830–834.

Morris, A. G. Conducting a parent education program in a pediatric clinic playroom. *Children Today*, 1974, 44, 11–14.

Mueller, E., & Vandell, D. Infant–infant interaction. In J. D. Osofsky (Ed.), *Handbook of Infant Development*. New York: Wiley, 1979.

Oremland, E. K., & Oremland, J. E. *The Effects of Hospitalization on Children*. Springfield, Illinois: Charles C Thomas, 1973.

Parten, M. Social participation among pre-school children. *Journal of Abnormal and Social Psychology*, 1932, 27, 243–269.

Petrillo, M. Guidelines for preoperative teaching. Unpublished material distributed at Utica College workshop, fall, 1978.

Petrillo, M. Preparing children and parents for hospitalization and treatment. *Pediatric Annals*, 1972, 1(3), 24–41.

Petrillo, M. & Sanger, S. *Emotional Care of Hospitalized Children.* Philadelphia: Lippincott, 1980.

Piaget, J. Piaget's theory. In P. H. Mussen (Ed.), *Carmichael's Manual of Child Psychology.* (3rd ed.) New York: Wiley, 1970.

Piaget, J. *Play, Dreams, and Imitation in Childhood.* New York: Norton, 1962.

Pickerill, C. M., & Pickerill, H. P. Elimination of hospital cross-infection in children: Nursing by the mother. *Lancet,* 1954, 266(1), 425–429.

Plank, E. N. *Working with Children in Hospitals.* Cleveland: Press of Case Western Reserve University, 1971.

Prugh, D. G., Staub, E., Sands, H. H., Kirschbaum, R. J., & Lenihan, E. A. A study of the emotional reactions of children and families to hospitalization and illness. *American Journal of Orthopsychiatry,* 1953, 23, 70–106.

Quinton, D., & Rutter, M. Early hospital admissions and later disturbances of behavior: An attempted replication of Douglas' findings. *Developmental Medicine and Child Neurology,* 1976, 18, 447–459.

Resnick, R., & Hergenroeder, E. Children in the emergency room. *Children Today,* 1975, 44, 5–8.

Robertson, J. *Young Children in Hospitals.* New York: Basic Books, 1958.

Rothenburg, M. B. Is there a national conspiracy against children in the United States? In Association for the Care of Children in Hospitals, *Human Needs and Political Realities.* Washington, D.C.: ACCH, no date.

Rubin, K. H., Maioni, T. L., & Hornung, M. Free play behaviors in middle- and lower-class preschoolers: Parten and Piaget revisited. *Child Development,* 1976, 47, 414–419.

Rutkowski, J. A survey of child life programs. *Journal of the Association for the Care of Children in Hospitals,* 1978, 6(4), 11–16.

Scarr-Salapatak, S., & Williams, M. L. The effects of early stimulation on low birth weight infants. *Child Development,* 1973, 44(1), 94–101.

Schaffer, H. R., & Callendar, W. J. Psychological effects of hospitalization in infancy. *Pediatrics,* 1959, 24, 528–539.

Skipper, J. K., & Leonard, R. C. Children, stress, and hospitalization: A field experiment. *Journal of Health and Social Behavior,* 1968, 9, 275–287.

Stanford, G. Now is the time: The professionalization of child life workers. *Journal of the Association for the Care of Children in Hospitals,* 1980, 8(3), 55–59.

Stanford, G. A survey to determine employment prospects for child life workers. Paper presented at the annual conference of the Association for the Care of Children in Hospitals, Los Angeles, 1979.

Umphenour, J. H. Bacterial colonization in neonates with sibling visitation. *Journal of Obstetric, Gynecologic and Neonatal Nursing,* 1980, 9(2), 73–75.

Vaughan, G. F. Children in hospital. *Lancet,* 1957, 272(2), 1117–1120.

Vernon, D. T. A., Foley, J. M., Sipowicz, R. R., & Schulman, J. L. *The Psychological Responses of Children to Hospitalization and Illness.* Springfield, Illinois: Charles C Thomas, 1965.

Vernon, D. T. A., Schulman, J. L., & Foley, J. M. Changes in children's behavior after hospitalization. *American Journal of the Diseases of Children,* 1966, 111, 581–593.

Weinick, H. M. Psychological study of emotional reactions of children to tonsillectomy. Unpublished doctoral dissertation, New York University, 1958.

Wolfer, J. A., & Visintainer, M. A. Pediatric surgical patients' and parents' stress responses and adjustment as a function of psychological preparation and stress-point nursing care. *Nursing Research*, 1975, 24(4), 244–255.

INDEX

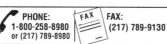 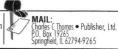